The Power of Ten

2011–2013

Nurse Leaders Address the Profession's Ten Most Pressing Issues

 Sigma Theta Tau International
Honor Society of Nursing

Sigma Theta Tau International

Copyright © 2011 by Sigma Theta Tau International

The Honor Society of Nursing, Sigma Theta Tau International (STTI) is a nonprofit organization whose mission is to support the learning, knowledge, and professional development of nurses committed to making a difference in health worldwide. Founded in 1922, STTI has 130,000 members in 86 countries. Members include practicing nurses, instructors, researchers, policymakers, entrepreneurs, and others. STTI's 470 chapters are located at 586 institutions of higher education throughout Australia, Botswana, Brazil, Canada, Colombia, Ghana, Hong Kong, Japan, Kenya, Malawi, Mexico, the Netherlands, Pakistan, Singapore, South Africa, South Korea, Swaziland, Sweden, Taiwan, Tanzania, the United States, and Wales. More information about STTI can be found online at *www.nursingsociety.org*.

Sigma Theta Tau International
550 West North Street
Indianapolis, IN 46202

To order additional books, buy in bulk, or order for corporate use, contact Nursing Knowledge International TOLL-FREE at 888.654.4968 (US and Canada) or +1.317.634.8171 (outside US and Canada).

To request a review copy for course adoption, e-mail solutions@nursingknowledge.org or call TOLL-FREE at 888.654.4968 (US and Canada) or +1.317.634.8171 (outside US and Canada).

To request author information, or for speaker or other media requests, contact Rachael McLaughlin of the Honor Society of Nursing, Sigma Theta Tau International at 888.634.7575 (US and Canada) or +1.317.634.8171 (outside US and Canada).

ISBN-13: 9781-935476-53-5
EPUB ISBN: 9781-935476-54-2
PDF ISBN: 9781-935476-55-9

Library of Congress Cataloging-in-Publication Data

Available from http://catalog.loc.gov/

Publisher: Renee Wilmeth
Acquisitions Editor: Janet Boivin, RN
Advisory Editor: Jim Mattson
Copy Editor and Indexer: Jane Palmer
Interior Design and
   Page Composition: Rebecca Batchelor

Principal Editor: Carla Hall
Development Editor: Renee Wilmeth
Project Editor: Katie Meyer
Editorial Coordinator: Paula Jeffers
Cover Design: Katy Bodenmiller

First Printing, 2011

Table of Contents

Preface

"What do you think are the 10 most important issues facing the nursing profession in the next 3 years?"

When we asked that question of prominent nurse leaders, we did not anticipate the number of responses, nor the care and passion of those who responded. So we decided to dig a little deeper, sorting and compiling the responses into categories and themes, and cross-checking our responses with major nurse surveys and reports, including the 2008 National Sample Survey of Registered Nurses and the Institute of Medicine's *The Future of Nursing: Leading Change, Advancing Health*.

When the information was pulled together, I was struck by the significance of the top 10 issues and their potential for reshaping health care and the nursing profession. Clearly, shifts in political and cultural climates, advances in technology, and changes in world demographics are giving nurses unprecedented opportunities to advance and strengthen the profession's role in global health care.

It was an easy decision for Sigma Theta Tau International to work with the respondents and other nursing leaders to craft a compelling, accessible, and thought-provoking book around these 10 powerful issues:

1. Evidence-Based Practice—Harmful or Helpful?
2. What Is the Impact of Technology on Nursing?

3. Nursing Education, Part I: Can We All Agree That a Bachelor's Degree Should Be the Minimum Level for Entry Into Practice?

4. Nursing Education, Part II: DNP vs. PhD—Separate but Equal?

5. How Do Nurses Get a Seat at the Policy Table?

6. How Do Nurses Cope With the Growing Ethical Demands of Practice?

7. How Do We Fix the Workplace Culture of Nursing?

8. What Role Do Nurse Leaders Play in the Profession?

9. What Are We Going to Do With This Widening Workforce Age Gap?

10. How Do We Make the Profession as Diverse as the Population for Which It Cares?

This book is for every nurse or nursing student who wants to understand the issues that are shaping the profession. We welcome all nurses across all levels and from all practice settings to join the conversation about these critical issues in nursing.

The nursing profession is at an historic crossroads. Never before have politicians, the public, and leaders of the health care industry recognized the importance of nurses' roles in preventing illness and injury and maintaining and improving the nation's health. It is up to us as nurses to use this opportunity to advance nursing's invaluable role in health care.

–Patricia E. Thompson, EdD, RN, FAAN
Chief Executive Officer
Honor Society of Nursing, Sigma Theta Tau International

Foreword

Health Care Transformation Needs Nurses to Succeed

American health care is in the midst of major social and economic upheaval, and it is clear the system that has evolved during the last 60 years is unsustainable. Transforming such a large and critical system will face political, personal, structural, and financial challenges.

Also clear is the fact that health care transformation will not be successful unless nurses participate in every phase of the change continuum. RNs make up the single largest component of clinical decision makers in the health care system and are located at the intersection of almost every patient care activity. Yet, the importance of their contribution to setting direction, forming policy, and building the structure of change is often given short shrift, despite rhetoric to the contrary.

Nursing leaders, be they organizational or clinical, must conceptualize the broad range of converging forces that directly influence the system's and the profession's competence in accurately and effectively addressing necessary change. Indeed, nurses must provide insightful leadership in transforming policy, infrastructure, and practice to configure a good fit between the demand for health service innovation and the collective response to that demand.

A number of historic issues impede a cohesive, informed nursing response to health transformation. These issues include BSN as minimal entry to the profession, clear differentiation of practice, fully practicing to one's scope of competence, regulatory inconsistencies across states, incongruous academic-service interface, and many other concerns that must be quickly resolved.

The profession must also confront an emerging digital context that affects every element of health service and nursing practice from this time forward. The growing interconnectedness between technology and the human experience challenges nurses to reconceptualize the foundations of practice and configure clinical modalities to reflect the integration of newer technologies. These technologies, reflected in value-driven practice, user engagement, evidentiary dynamics, human simulation, comparative effectiveness research, interdisciplinary integration, and seamless documentation along the health continuum, all serve to reformat health care delivery and nursing practice.

This book, *The Power of Ten, 2011-2013: Nurse Leaders Address the Profession's Ten Most Pressing Issues*, demonstrates the authors' recognition of these shifting realities and the issues that reflect them. Within the pages of this book, the reader will find critical insights addressing a broad range of the relevant issues and suggested actions that may help to better align dynamic and emerging realities with appropriate responses.

The content provides a timely synthesis of critical thinking and possible responses that helps position nursing leadership to undertake thoughtful and informed action. Time is of the essence; information is critical, and action is the requisite. With the insights contained in this book, nurse leaders have what they need to appropriately and fully engage the creative act of building a truly effective American health care system.

–Tim Porter-O'Grady, DM, EdD, FAAN
Senior Partner, Tim Porter-O'Grady Associates, Inc.
Registered Medical Mediator, Health Systems Consultation
Atlanta, Georgia

Associate Professor, Leadership Scholar
Program in Health Innovation, CONHI
Arizona State University
Phoenix, Arizona

Visiting Professor, DNP Program
University of Maryland School of Nursing
Baltimore, Maryland

Introduction

In December 2009, I asked Jim Mattson, our longtime editor of *Reflections on Nursing Leadership (RNL)*, to prepare a report for our STTI publications team. The topic? "What are the top 10 issues facing the profession in the next 3 years?" Of course, my ulterior motive was hoping Jim's thoughts would spur discussion at our semi-annual publications brainstorming meeting that leads to book ideas.

Jim sent out e-mails to many of his top contacts with RNL, and imagine my surprise when he arrived at the meeting with an amazing array of answers from at least 30 nurse leaders and educators from around the world, many of whom are names you will recognize. And while I was amazed at the response, what really struck me was how consistently similar the responses were. While each issue is a topic that is often controversial and causes great debate among leaders, here were 30 people from widely varying backgrounds, practices, and locations with similar ideas. The impact was staggering.

After a spirited discussion internally, we realized that these topics were a book in and of themselves. Do we expect you to agree with everything presented? Of course not. And we've been purposefully provocative in some cases. Our purpose with this book is to get a discussion going. If you have the same reaction we did, it becomes more difficult to sweep some of these debates aside—hoping that someone else will take them up. We think it's time for the nursing profession to start the conversation!

We have designed the book for self-study or for a group. Try gathering your colleagues and discussing each issue over lunch once a month. Try researching issues you're not familiar with, and voice your own recommendations for change. Make notes in the book. Mark it up. If something makes you a little mad, take advantage of that passion. Being passionate about a topic means you can advocate for change! Get really riled up? Or want to discuss more with other readers? Come check our website—www.powerof10book.org—and join the conversation!

–*Renee Wilmeth*
Publisher
Sigma Theta Tau International

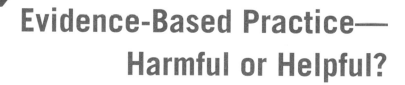

Question #1:

Evidence-Based Practice— Harmful or Helpful?

Did you know…

Evidence-based practice, in its simplest form, means using evidence to guide practice (Dickerson, 2010).

Evidence-based practice (EBP) isn't exactly a new idea. Florence Nightingale used statistical analysis to measure outcomes, and it's been argued by scholars that she was one of its first proponents. It's been much discussed, studied, and researched and today is as close to a ubiquitous gold standard as nursing may ever have.

But experts are starting to wonder what the long-term effects of EBP will be on patient care and the ability of nurses to deliver it. Improving patient care is the prime directive, and while EBP systematically improves outcomes, nurses are starting to wonder if they will ever have time to fluff a pillow again. Best practices and efficacy are great—especially if you're in charge of the bottom line—but the time you take to reassure a patient's husband or wife can make a real difference in discharge rates.

To be more academic about it, nurses employ critical thinking every day as they assess patients and consider what the patient needs. Looking at the total patient *as well as* the evidence and protocol is essential. However, within the parameters of EBP, where is the room for creativity? Where is the permission to look at patient needs? Will a desire for more quantifiable outcomes prevent a nurse from taking the time to do the most important thing—be a nurse?

There is no question that nursing is better off with EBP, but have you considered the positives and negatives of EBP in your own practice? Do you see it improving over time? If not, maybe it's time to start the conversation.

Evidence-Based Practice: Hard Work But Worth It

by Maureen Dobbins

Sir Muir Gray, a pioneer in evidence-based practice (EBP), told me a few years ago that the application of what we currently know will have a bigger impact on health and disease than any drug or technology likely to be delivered in the next decade. This statement empowers every health care professional—including nurses—from point-of-care to policy development, to consider the role they have to play in ensuring that what we know works in health care is identified from the best quality research evidence, and is integrated into policy and practice decisions.

EBP was identified in a recent survey as one of the 10 most important issues facing the nursing profession. This is a call to action and provides much-needed recognition of the importance of putting into practice what works, and furthermore eliminating those practices we know do not work.

A senior decision maker indicated recently that EBP is devilishly hard work. We also know that EBP is not an individual sport, but rather requires a unified and orchestrated team effort. While individual roles to support, implement, and maintain EBP differ depending on one's position and responsibility in an organization, we must all endeavor to play our part. At the bedside, nurses must strive to be continuously open to changing practice based on emerging new knowledge, keeping in mind the goal of ensuring optimal health for our patients and clients.

What do you think?
_____

_____

_____

_____

_____

_____

_____

_____

_____

discussion point

Does evidence-based practice decrease a nurse's ability to determine care based on how she sees a patient respond?

_____

_____

_____

_____

_____

_____

_____

Nurse managers must be open to look at all the research evidence evaluating a particular intervention; identify those that are effective as well as those that are not; and determine the feasibility and acceptability of those interventions in different contexts. Furthermore, nurse managers must work collaboratively with those at the bedside to eliminate ineffective interventions from practice.

At the organizational level, we need strong senior leadership, both nursing and otherwise, to support, cultivate, enable, and expect EBP at all levels of the organization. This is not a short and easy jog down the street, but rather a multiyear journey requiring dedicated resources, both human and financial, to develop the knowledge, attitudes, skill, capacity, and culture to practice in an evidence-based way. Changes at all levels are needed starting with the organization itself and trickling down over time to divisions, teams, and individual nurses. There are some excellent examples of EBP with positive patient outcomes.

While EBP requires significant upfront investment, the long-term gains in improved patient and population health outcomes are worth the effort. The time has come to join together as a profession to ensure that we practice every day, to the best of our ability, in an evidence-based way.

–Maureen Dobbins, _PhD, RN, is associate professor, School of Nursing, cross-appointed with the Department of Epidemiology and Biostatistics and the School of Rehabilitation Sciences, McMaster University, Hamilton, Ontario, Canada._

The Future of Evidence-Based Practice: From Goal to Reality

by Bernadette Mazurek Melnyk

Although it is now well-recognized that evidence-based practice (EBP) enhances the quality of care, improves patient outcomes, and reduces health care costs, it is not routinely implemented by clinicians and is not the standard of practice in many health care systems across the United States.

"Nursing research and practice must continue to identify and develop evidence-based improvements to care, and these improvements must be tested and adopted through policy changes across the health care system"
(Institute of Medicine, 2011).

Top 10 challenges

"What have educators done to nurses? We espouse evidence-based care—yes, we need to—but is this at the expense of a much greater fundamental requirement? What happens to the 10% (or whatever) who do not respond to an intervention? What has happened to the human factor? Sometimes I feel that hairdressers give better psychological care than nurses. They give advice from the heart without the worry of the big question, 'Is this what research tells us?' We still need to value clinical judgment, human contact, and gut reaction."

–Angela Kydd, PhD, MSc, RGN, RMN, PGCE, senior lecturer in gerontology, School of Health, Nursing and Midwifery at the University of the West of Scotland

Top 10 challenges

"EBP informs our practice but is not the only way to practice, because we are working with individuals, not numbers."

–Claudia K.Y. Lai, PhD, RN, professor, Hong Kong Polytechnic University School of Nursing, Hong Kong SAR, China

Unfortunately, the translation of findings from research into clinical practice often takes several years, and—for many studies—the results are never translated into clinical practice to improve care. In order to accelerate EBP, the Institute of Medicine set a goal that, by 2020, 90% of health care decisions will be evidence-based. However, this goal will only be realized when:

1. Health care systems make it their mission to deliver evidence-based care and invest resources in creating sustainable cultures of EBP.

2. Educational institutions teach baccalaureate and master's degree students how to take an evidence-based approach to care, instead of how to conduct the rigorous process of research.

3. Clinicians develop the knowledge and skills necessary to consistently deliver evidence-based care.

4. Evidence is generated to guide practices where it is lacking.

5. Best practices are integrated into information technology systems.

6. Leaders and managers model evidence-based decision-making.

7. Health care systems and clinicians are routinely incentivized to deliver EBP.

Top 10 challenges

"I'm concerned about the backlash of evidence-based practice as it pushes out and dampens innovation and creativity."

–Daniel J. Pesut, PhD, RN, PMHCNS-BC, FAAN, past president of STTI,
professor and associate dean for graduate programs,
Indiana University School of Nursing, Indianapolis, Indiana, USA

discussion point

Have you been in a situation where you felt a patient's outcome suffered at the hands of EBP?

EBP is a seven-step, problem-solving approach to the delivery of health care that integrates the best evidence from a body of studies with a clinician's expertise and a patient's preferences and values. Important components of clinical expertise in the EBP paradigm include data gathered from a thorough patient assessment; internal evidence generated from outcomes management, quality improvement initiatives, and EBP implementation projects; and the evaluation of and use of available resources necessary to achieve desired patient outcomes.

Although external evidence generated from research creates a solid foundation upon which to base clinical practice, there are many areas of patient care in which rigorous research is not available to guide informed practice decisions. When external evidence is not available, clinicians must consistently generate internal evidence to guide their practices.

Top 10 challenges

"We need continued advancement in evidence-based practice to continue to move our profession forward."

–Vicki Michelle McMahon, MSN, RN

Top 10 challenges

"Hospitals and organizations should provide more support for evidence-based practice at the staff nurse level. Certainly, they should be involved in establishing policies, etc., but they don't have the time to do all the research and investigation that some hospitals are asking them to do."

–Cynthia Saver, MS, RN, president of CLS Development, Inc., Columbia, Maryland, USA

The barriers to EBP are well-documented. These include nurses' perception that it takes too much time, lack of administrative support and tools to support evidence-based care, and negative attitudes toward research that are, in large part, a result of how educational programs have taught research over the years. We are at a point where we no longer need to focus on EBP barriers as we know them. In order to advance EBP, we now need to invest in research-based facilitators of EBP that include building cultures of EBP, using EBP mentors who work with front-line clinicians in implementing EBP, and providing clinicians with the EBP knowledge, skills, and tools they need to consistently deliver evidence-based care.

Academic curriculums need to be redesigned to prepare clinicians who are equipped to implement EBP and transform health care cultures. Faculties in academic institutions also need to gain EBP skills, because they cannot teach students what they themselves do not know. Further, consumers must be educated on how their health outcomes will improve with evidence-based care and encouraged to demand it from their health care providers. Finally, more research on the best strategies to advance EBP is needed. Only when these tactics are executed across the United States will the IOM 2020 goal become a reality.

–Bernadette Mazurek Melnyk, *PhD, RN, CPNP/PMHNP, FNAP, FAAN, is current dean and Distinguished Foundation Professor of Nursing at the Arizona State University College of Nursing & Health Innovation and incoming associate vice president for health promotion, chief wellness officer, and dean of the College of Nursing at The Ohio State University.*

Did you know…

More than 150 years before the landmark Institute of Medicine (IOM) reports on quality of health care (*To Err Is Human: Building a Safer Health System*, 1999; *Crossing the Quality Chasm*, 2001; and nine additional reports in the *IOM Quality Chasm* series) created a flurry of EBP initiatives, Florence Nightingale, the founder of modern nursing, was practicing EBP to great success.

> *In her quest to improve the conditions of hospitals during the Crimean War, Nightingale assessed the environment, collected data, identified interventions and monitored patient outcomes. In less than six months her interventions significantly decreased the mortality of soldiers who were dying from wounds, infections, cholera and lack of adequate care. Nightingale utilized supporting evidence to transform healthcare (Cooper, n.d., para. 2).*

In addition to everything else she did, Florence Nightingale was also an early pioneer of presenting information visually. Early pie charts were, at the time, a relatively novel method of presenting data. Nightingale used them to show relationships of data to improve health (Wikipedia, n.d.).

"Although it is difficult to prove causation, an emerging body of literature suggests that quality of care depends to a large degree on nurses" (Institute of Medicine, 2011, p. 26).

EBP at the Bedside

by Stephanie Poe

The role of evidence-based practice (EBP) at the bedside and across health care settings remains one of the most vital issues in nursing today. The Institute of Medicine (IOM) recently released a groundbreaking publication that presents unprecedented opportunity and challenge for the nursing profession and highlights the importance of EBP (IOM, 2011). This timely report presents a thought-provoking vision of the future of nursing, with nurses as full partners and innovative leaders in improving health care and the complex system in which care is delivered. It advocates for nurses to practice to the full extent of their education and training, with the goal of achieving patient care of the highest quality.

All health professionals share a core set of competencies that are directed toward the goals of delivering patient-centered care, employing quality improvement principles, working in interdisciplinary teams, *applying evidence-based practices*, and using health information technologies (IOM, 2003). The ability to ask important practice questions, analyze and synthesize the best available evidence, and translate this evidence into practice is critical to the transformation of nurses into full partners in co-creating the future of health care. Using an EBP approach assures that nurses have access to state-of-the art strategies to make good decisions. Such access increases the likelihood of achieving quality outcomes, augments the credibility of nursing decisions in the eyes of professional colleagues, and enhances meaningful interdisciplinary collaboration and care coordination.

This unparalleled opportunity presents considerable challenges to the nursing profession. The needs of patients, families, and communities are dynamic, and nursing practice is continually evolving, adapting, and transforming to meet the nation's health requirements. The economic climate is characterized by increased competition for scarce resources. The need for and value of allocating time and opportunity for nurses to participate in EBP are often underappreciated. These challenges are real, but not insurmountable.

As stewards of the largest component of the health care workforce, nurse leaders are well positioned to combine the art and science of nursing to build a culture of nursing excellence. Their role in setting the vision, creating a supportive infrastructure for building competence in EBP, and facilitating the conduct of nurse-led EBP projects has the potential to advance nursing practice, improve patient outcomes, and promote the nurse's role in clinical decision making. A commitment to EBP enables nurse leaders to help transform the health care system to meet the demand for safe, quality, accessible, affordable, patient-centered care.

–**Stephanie Poe, DNP, RN,** *is director of nursing, clinical quality, and chief nursing information officer at The Johns Hopkins Hospital, Baltimore, Maryland, with a joint appointment with The Johns Hopkins University School of Nursing.*

**It's your turn...
start the discussion!**

References

Cooper, C. (n.d.). Transforming health care through the use of evidence-based practice. *Nursing Excellence, 1*(1). Retrieved from http://www.childrenscentralcal.org/PRESSROOM/PUBLICATIONS/NX1/Pages/NX-V1-I1-A2.aspx

Dickerson, P.S. (2010). *Evidence-based practice: Why does it matter?* Retrieved from http://www.healthcaretodayonline.com/HCTclassroom/coursematerials0610.pdf

Institute of Medicine. (2003). *Health professions education: A bridge to quality.* Washington, DC: The National Academies Press.

Institute of Medicine. (2011). *The future of nursing: Leading change, advancing health.* Washington, DC: The National Academies Press.

Wikipedia. (n.d.) *Florence Nightingale.* Retrieved from http://en.wikipedia.org/wiki/Florence_Nightingale#Nursing

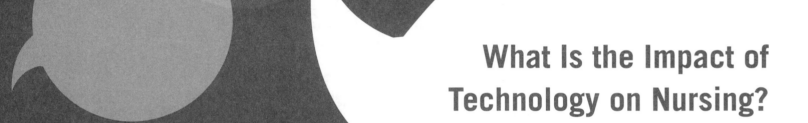

Question #2:

What Is the Impact of Technology on Nursing?

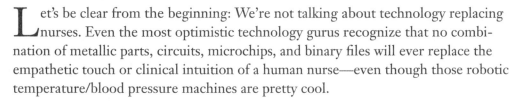

"Nurses [need] to understand that technology is here to stay; we need to embrace it and work to be sure it serves us instead of us serving it."

–Cynthia Saver, *MS, RN, president of CLS Development, Inc., Columbia, Maryland, USA*

Let's be clear from the beginning: We're not talking about technology replacing nurses. Even the most optimistic technology gurus recognize that no combination of metallic parts, circuits, microchips, and binary files will ever replace the empathetic touch or clinical intuition of a human nurse—even though those robotic temperature/blood pressure machines are pretty cool.

What we *are* talking about is the ongoing integration of technology into your daily practice. There's no question that technology improves health care, but what nursing professionals have to figure out is how technology also changes the patient experience. It's one thing to calm patients at the bedside, but something else entirely to calm them from behind an electronic charting tablet or computer screen.

As nurses, it's time to start the conversation about how we can embrace technology while not losing sight of our humanity. From electronic health care records to patient simulators, advanced technological systems will continue to be a major part of the patient experience. Are you going to be dedicated to finding new ways to integrate the technology into your daily practice? What role can you play in not only improving health care, but also improving *patient care?* The answer may be to ensure that the best patient advocates—nurses—are at the table when decisions are made about the design, development, and implementation of new technologies.

But that's just the beginning. When nurses *do* make it to the planning process, they need to know (and understand) what the technology is and its implications. Most importantly, nurses have a momentous opportunity to become true advocates for their patients. When using certain technologies that could erect psychological walls between nurses and patients, it is up to nurses to speak up when they sense that these patients feel as though they're being treated like a robot: just another machine to be scanned, probed, tuned or adjusted.

To Err Is Human, To EHR Is to Minimize Errors

by Manuel C. Co Jr.

Advances in clinical care and public health have contributed to people living longer. With greater life expectancy, individuals with chronic conditions such as high blood pressure, high cholesterol, diabetes, and asthma are now being managed in ambulatory care, the community, and the patient's own home. Similarly, advances in information and communication technology (ICT) blending audiovisual and telephone with computer networks have resulted in their ubiquitous use in an increasingly urban and more globally connected community.

The challenges we are facing include the burden of chronic and noncommunicable diseases, the threat of epidemics and pandemics, the rising costs of health care, and the quality chasm that still exists between the ideal care and the care that is provided. To address these, we must develop and maintain better information infrastructure to provide the backbone for supporting population-based care outcomes.

discussion point

Do you think technology versus patient care is an "either/or" situation? If you had to assign a percentage value to each component, what would it be and why?

Did you know …

"Even though there was talk about using computers in medicine as technology advanced in the early twentieth century, it was not until the 1950s that informatics really took off in the United States. Robert Ledley, who would later invent the first full body CT scanner, is often credited as one of the founding fathers of U.S. informatics. His use of computers in dental projects with the National Bureau of Standards set the stage for later advancements in applying information technology to medicine."

(University of Illinois at Chicago, n.d., para. 2)

We can start with an interdisciplinary approach to understand and integrate clinicians' workflow into the design of an electronic health record (EHR) and to minimize any error potential by learning from published studies on its unintended consequences. Special attention to the usability of technology as applied to a particular care setting will ensure that nurses and other health care team members find it usable and useful to their practice. In the case of using ICT as a health intervention tool, the participant's health literacy level needs to be considered when designing interactive user interfaces.

Although the presence of comprehensive and/or fully functional EHRs is concentrated in larger institutions, such as academic and teaching hospitals and larger physician group practices, we can expect higher EHR adoption across care settings, given the Medicare incentive payments for eligible hospitals and eligible professionals for adoption, implementation, upgrade, or demonstration of meaningful use of certified EHR technology based on specified objectives and measures.

Top 10 challenges

"[The problem can be] becoming infatuated with technology to the extent that it distracts us from understanding larger principles and practice."

—**Sarah H. Kagan**, PhD, RN, Lucy Walker Honorary Term Professor of Gerontological Nursing and clinical nurse specialist, Abramson Cancer Center, University of Pennsylvania, USA

We must include standards-based use of data elements to support interoperability, defined as the ability of EHRs to work together within and across organizational boundaries, for exchanging patient health information. Doing so enhances care coordination and enables data aggregation to lend insights on the health care delivery and outcomes being measured.

Finally, data in EHRs must reflect nursing's holistic perspective and capture nursing's contributions to care outcomes, and nurses need to embrace direct patient use of ICT as an extension of their nursing practice.

This is an exciting opportunity to collaborate in developing information infrastructure. There is no better time to do this than now!

Acknowledgment: Special thanks to Dr. Suzanne Bakken of Columbia University for her thoughtful feedback to my manuscript draft.

—**Manuel C. Co Jr.,** *MSN, MS, RN, CPHIMS, is a predoctoral fellow and Jonas Scholar at Columbia University School of Nursing and adjunct informatics faculty at Hunter-Bellevue School of Nursing, Hunter College, City University of New York, USA.*

"[An important issue is] the changing nature of learning in nursing with the incorporation of simulation and social media and technology."

–**Daniel J. Pesut,** *PhD, RN, PMHCNS-BC, FAAN, professor, Indiana University School of Nursing, Indianapolis, Indiana, USA*

"Technology has the potential to either humanize or dehumanize care, enhance or interfere with professional scope of practice, interdisciplinary partnership and clinical integration. It can ensure evidence-based practice or lead to institutional, task-driven practice. It has the potential to transform education of nursing students and bridge the gap between the desired practice reality and the inadequate present-day institutional realities lived at the point of care. It has the ability to assure that health care, not just medical care, will be available for this society."

–Bonnie Wesorick, *MSN, RN, FAAN, founder, CPM Resource Center, Grand Rapids, Michigan, USA*

Did you know…

"The TIGER Initiative (Technology Informatics Guiding Education Reform) is working to help the United States realize its 10-year goal of electronic health records for all its citizens. TIGER, which started as a grass-roots initiative, now involves more than 70 professional nursing organizations, vendors, and governmental entities.

"The TIGER Initiative aims to enable practicing nurses and nursing students to fully engage in the unfolding digital electronic era in healthcare. The purpose of the initiative is to identify information/knowledge management best practices and effective technology capabilities for nurses. TIGER's goal is to create and disseminate local and global action plans that can be duplicated within nursing and other multidisciplinary health care training and workplace settings." (The TIGER Initiative, n.d.)

Informatics: Using the Power of the Web to Empower Health Care

by Connie White Delaney

Nursing and other health professionals have a social mandate to serve the world's population, which was 6,924,848,096, according to the U.S. Census Bureau's World Population Clock, at the time this book went to press (June 14, 2011). We have closed the first decade of the 21st century and have experienced many driving forces of change, including scientific advancements, new synergies in information and communication technologies (ICT), and a near global imperative for containing health care costs and increasing quality, safety, and access. The future calls for intense integration of biomedical health informatics within a person-centered care delivery model, which encompasses population health, self-management in chronic disease, consumer empowerment, home as the central care location, and personalized care through genomics.

Top 10 challenges

"[We should] use technology wisely and effectively to promote nursing and health care."

–**Cynthia Clark**, PhD, RN, ANEF, professor of nursing, Boise State University, Idaho, USA

discussion point

How you integrate technology into patient care makes a difference. Identify three situations involving technology in your daily practice where you integrated a bedside or personal element into patient care.

"[We should] integrate informatics in all that we do."

–Michelle R. Troseth, *MSN, RN, DPNAP, executive vice president and chief professional practice officer, Elsevier*

According to AMIA (n.d.), biomedical and health informatics applies principles of computer and information science to the advancement of life sciences research, health professions education, public health, and patient care. This multidisciplinary and integrative field focuses on health information and communication technologies (HICT) and involves computer, cognitive, and social sciences. This interdisciplinary and diverse field:

- Combines health sciences (such as medicine, dentistry, nursing, pharmacy, and allied health) with computer science, management and decision science, biostatistics, engineering, and information technology.

- Solves problems in health care delivery; pharmaceutical, biomedical and health sciences research; and health education and clinical/medical decision making.

- Is essential in all aspects of health care and biomedicine.

Consequently, informatics is fundamental to nursing and all health care professions, and the future of health care; biomedical, clinical, and translational research; and public health.

Informatics is a critical foundation to all aspects of nursing's future, including research/scholarship, clinical practice, education, and leadership. Informatics focuses on nursing data and information, defining what should and could be collected, how to analyze it, and how it should be used to promote greater efficiency and effectiveness of health care and improve the population's health. Informatics is key to redefining Internet-empowered, "informed patient," and health consumerism leading to redefining the power relationship between patient and clinician toward that of "equal partner" in decision-making and care management.

Health and nursing informatics, both as essential competencies (Technology Informatics Guiding Educational Reform [The TIGER Initiative, n.d.]) for all professionals and as specialty preparation at the master's and doctoral level in nursing or health informatics, empowers all missions of the nursing profession. Informatics has become a vital component of nursing accreditation (e.g., Commission on Collegiate Nursing Education [CCNE], National League for Nursing [NLN]), and National Institute for Nursing Research [NINR, n.d.]).

The immense and extensive developments of nursing and health informatics have set the stage for dramatic and revolutionary changes in nursing and health care—a 21st century synergy. Truly, the tipping point has been reached where our discussions on whether there is a role for informatics in nursing practice, education, and research will be an everyday reality and remembered only as a bookmark in nursing's history.

—**Connie White Delaney,** *PhD, RN, FAAN, FACMI, is professor and dean, University of Minnesota School of Nursing; Academic Health Center, director, Biomedical Health Informatics (BMHI); associate director, CTSI/BMI; and acting director, Institute for Health Informatics (IHI).*

"[We are] becoming infatuated with technology to the extent that it distracts us from understanding larger principles and practice (e.g., high fidelity simulation is all 'of the moment,' but we miss that we have been simulating practice experiences for years in the name of education)."

–**Sarah H. Kagan,** *PhD, RN, Lucy Walker Honorary Term Professor of Gerontological Nursing and clinical nurse specialist, Abramson Cancer Center, University of Pennsylvania, USA*

"[An important issue is] the use and integration of simulation in nurse education. I facilitated the inaugural meeting of a European Network of Nurse Educators to try and share best practice. I held the second meeting of this group on 4 June 2011 in Granada, Spain. We had over 40 delegates from all across Europe, and we are now looking to affiliate this group with the International Nursing Association for Clinical Simulation and Learning (INACSL)."

–**Matthew Aldridge,** BSc (Hons) *Clinical Nursing Practice, MA (Ed), RN, Registered Nurse Teacher, FHEA, senior lecturer in acute adult nursing, University of Wolverhampton*

Technology: Transforming Nursing and Health Care

by Joyce Sensmeier

Nurses play an important role in leveraging health information technology (IT) to improve patient safety, quality, and efficiency of care delivery. The nursing workflow is complex, which poses challenges for the adoption of technology.

Nurses are essential for achieving quality outcomes through the implementation of electronic health record (EHR) systems. Deployment of technology is not simply the result of a decision about software and hardware. Instead, technology adoption should address areas that need improvement, thus leading an organization toward clinical transformation. Nurses have the right competencies and skills to drive these changes in the clinical setting, and their leadership is a necessary component for achieving success.

Nurses can also play an important role in helping patients understand and navigate emerging electronic tools such as personal health records (PHR) or patient portals. Ease of use and accessibility are essential for consumer engagement, and nurses should encourage their health care organizations to invest in user-friendly, secure portals and standards-based PHR systems. As technology becomes more pervasive, nurses should be advocates of these new avenues for engaging patients in acquiring credible information and gaining knowledge.

Nurses must also prepare themselves to practice in new and innovative ways. Future practice models may require a shift in roles and responsibilities where patients are active and knowledgeable partners, working together with their care providers in a technology-enhanced practice environment. Nurses must develop the necessary informatics competencies and act upon these new information management demands. Successfully acquiring these skills and embedding them in nursing practice will also enable patients to achieve their health goals and improve their quality of life.

"[One issue is] the challenge of balancing technology (robotics, simulation, etc.) and the human element."

–Carol L. Huston, *DPA, MSN, MPA, FAAN, director, School of Nursing, California State University, Chico, California, USA*

Top 10 challenges

"Nurses need to understand that technology is here to stay; we need to embrace it and work to be sure it serves us instead of us serving it."

–Cynthia Saver, MS, RN, president of CLS Development, Inc.

Today, most health records are stored in multiple locations, maintained by multiple providers, and recorded in both paper and electronic format. This lack of interoperability compounds our ability to ensure accuracy or availability of the information, thereby compromising health care quality. Nurses are active participants in most transitions of care, intuitively bridging information gaps where technology or processes may not support workflow. Often, the concepts of data

Did you know …

"On February 17, 2009, President Barack Obama signed into law the American Recovery and Reinvestment Act (ARRA). Title XIII of ARRA, called the Health IT for Economic and Clinical Health Act (HITECH), allocated $19.2 billion toward health IT. This act seeks to bolster health IT to improve the delivery of healthcare in the United States. With various provisions and regulations, the Act provides assistance, tools, and resources to providers to allow for implementation and utilization of electronic health records." (HIMSS, n.d.)

standards and health information exchange are viewed as too complex. However, nurses must be savvy enough to advocate for information systems that deliver the right information, about the right patient, at the right time, and in the right location.

As we look to the future, nurses can work with their informatics colleagues and leverage technology to transform the way they deliver care. Including nursing workflow as a focus of technology adoption will ensure that systems and devices enable nurses to be more efficient and ultimately improve health care quality.

—**Joyce Sensmeier,** *MS, RN-BC, CPHIMS, FHIMSS, FAAN, is vice president of informatics, HIMSS.*

Beyond Technology: Making Machines the Servants of Health Care

by Bonnie Wesorick

I believe the most urgent issue facing nursing today is health care reform, related to the use and impact of technology on practice and education. The federal authorities, supported by the American Reinvestment and Recovery Act Stimulus Package, have targeted financial incentives with meaningful use criteria to ensure that implementation of technology becomes a reality as part of health care reform.

Implementation of technology is at the core of health care reform, and if nursing is not at the table where decisions are being made related to policy, structure, design, development, and implementation of technology, both those who give and receive care will be at risk. This fast-paced federal program calls for nursing leadership at a level of intensity rarely experienced.

Technology has the potential to either humanize or dehumanize care, and either enhance or interfere with professional scope of practice, interdisciplinary partnership, and clinical integration. It can ensure evidence-based practice or lead to institutional and task-driven practice. It has the potential to transform the education of nursing students and bridge the gap between the desired practice

"[An important issue is] Informatics in nursing, especially what is meaningful use in terms of health information technology. Embedded in this are the issues of nursing knowledge classification systems and ways to standardize nursing knowledge—to get a meta thesaurus of standardized terms. There is great debate: We have NANDA, NIC, NOC in the US, and others are looking at the International Classification of Nursing Practice (ICNP) model that is being pushed by the ICN."

—**Daniel J. Pesut,** *PhD, RN, PMHCNS-BC, FAAN, professor, Indiana University School of Nursing, Indianapolis, Indiana, USA*

It's your turn ... start the discussion!

————————————————
————————————————
————————————————
————————————————
————————————————
————————————————
————————————————
————————————————
————————————————
————————————————

reality and the inadequate present-day institutional realities lived at the point of care. It has the ability to ensure that health care—not just medical care—will be available to our society.

The national agenda for health care reform will either advance nursing or limit it. Nursing's leadership is essential—not as a fight for power, but to ensure that the voice and wisdom of the largest group of health care professionals are present to help create a transformed health care system.

—**Bonnie Wesorick,** *MSN, RN, FAAN, is founder, CPM Resource Center, Grand Rapids, Michigan, USA.*

"I think that in Sweden and the rest of the European Union—maybe also the USA—one aspect of nursing and medicine will be increasingly important within the next couple of years. Person-centered care or patient-centered care is, according to the national GPCC (University of Gothenburg Centre for Person-Centered Care) center in Sweden, both a highly prioritized and essential aspect of the health care structure. In nursing, the questions and discussion should, therefore, target both person-centered care as a more theoretic core as well as the specific nursing aspect within this area. One area that I think would be interesting to illuminate is the need for more person-centered e-health/telemedicine. Another area is how social media can be a tool in the clinic of tomorrow."

–Axel Wolf, *MSc, RN, CRNA, PhD student, The Sahlgrenska Academy, Göteborg University, Göteborg, Sweden*

References

AMIA. (n.d.). *About AMIA*. Retrieved from https://www.amia.org/inside

HIMSS. (n.d.) *Legislation and regulations*. Retrieved from http://himss.org/ASP/topics_FocusDynamic.
asp?faid=402

National Institute of Nursing Research. (n.d.). *Mission & strategic plan*. Retrieved from http://www.ninr.nih.
gov/AboutNINR/NINRMissionandStrategicPlan

The TIGER Initiative. (n.d.). *About TIGER*. Retrieved from http://www.tigersummit.com/About_Us.html

U.S. Census Bureau. (2011). *U.S. & world population clocks*. Retrieved from http://www.census.gov/main/
www/popclock.html

University of Illinois at Chicago. (n.d.). *The history of health informatics*. Retrieved from http://healthinfor-
matics.uic.edu/history-of-health-informatics

Question #3:

Nursing Education, Part I: Can We All Agree That a Bachelor's Degree Should Be the Minimum Level for Entry Into Practice?

"[An important issue is] failure of nursing to maintain an education entry level similar to that of the other health care professions."

–**Carol L. Huston**, *DPA, MSN, MPA, FAAN, director, School of Nursing, California State University, Chico, California, USA*

Hey, it's a controversial statement. You probably work with qualified and excellent colleagues who themselves might not be what we loftily call "bachelor's-prepared." So, it's hard to think about the terrific nurses who might not make it into practice if we were to say "BSNs only."

But think of it this way: Without requiring BSN preparation for nurses—a minimum qualification for most professionals—how can we demand professional status ourselves? Physical, speech, and occupational therapies all require a master's degree for entry into practice. Nursing is no less complex. One could argue that nurses require more knowledge and expertise because they are dealing with the entire human body and mind—not just one particular aspect. So what gives? What will it take to commit to making a bachelor's degree the minimum level for entry into nursing practice?

The primary arguments against the BSN requirement for nurses involve time and money. But with most students already committing to an associate's degree nursing program that takes 2 to 3 years to complete, does 1 or 2 more years of critical training create a hardship? College education in any field is expensive, but that extra time can provide crucial training and knowledge for a successful career. (How about we start to combat that turnover rate for new nursing grads?) College is expensive. So, why should nursing students be any different?

Are we oversimplifying the issue to make a point? Of course. But let's start the discussion.

Minimum Education Levels for Nursing Professionals: Decades of Debate, Still No Resolution in Sight

by Carol Huston

Minimum educational levels for entry into practice in nursing have been debated since the 1940s, and a now infamous 1965 position paper by the American Nurses Association suggested the need for an orderly transition from hospital-based diploma nursing preparation to nursing education in colleges or universities.

Now, 46 years later, despite intermittent passionate debate, increasing scope and complexity of professional nursing roles, and new and compelling evidence linking the educational preparation of nurses and patient outcomes, limited progress has been made in achieving this goal. While the majority of nurses in the United States are no longer educated in diploma programs, they are educated at an associate's degree (community college) level.

Clearly, registered nurses have resisted the normal course of occupational development that other health care professions have pursued. As a result, nurses are now the least educated health care professionals, with most health care professions requiring master's and doctoral degrees for entry. Indeed, one must question whether nursing could or should lose its designation as a profession because of its failure to maintain educational equity. The primary identity of any professional

discussion point

Do you have a bachelor's or more advanced degree? Do your colleagues? Do you think a bachelor's degree should be a minimum requirement for entry into nursing practice? Why or why not?

Did you know ...

The Institute of Medicine's 2011 report, *The Future of Nursing: Leading Change, Advancing Health*, makes it clear that education is one of the four key messages nurses need to carry forward into the future. But, the report puts the responsibility on both the student and educational system: "Nurses should achieve higher levels of education and training through an improved education system that promotes seamless academic progression." Authors of the report acknowledge that we are not there yet.

"Major changes in the U.S. health care system and practice environment will require equally profound changes in the education of nurses both before and after they receive their licenses." (Institute of Medicine, 2011)

group is based at least in part on established educational entry level. How can nursing argue that education is unimportant and makes no difference in how we practice or the outcomes that result?

Complicating the picture is the fact that 2-year Associate Degrees in Nursing (ADN) now take three or four years to complete, and the content differentiation that Mildred Montag, a leader in the field of ADN education, originally described regarding university and technical nursing programs does not exist. Many ADN programs have added content traditionally reserved for baccalaureate education, such as leadership, management, research, and community health. As a result, their graduates often feel short-changed when awarded a technical degree. In addition, RNs who return to school for a university degree often encounter limited integration, standardization, or cooperation between public systems of education; duplicative learning; and high tuition costs that have no promise of fiduciary payoff in future employment.

The end result is that 7 decades after the debate began, entry into practice continues to be hotly debated, with little resolution in sight. Can we all agree that a BSN should be the minimum level for entry into practice? I believe that will not happen until special interests can be put aside in favor of an objective analysis of what education is needed for 21st century nurses and for the safety of the public we serve. It will only happen when an educational system is in place that allows seamless, integrated educational advancement for RNs who want to return to school.

—**Carol Huston**, *DPA, MSN, MPA, FAAN, is director of the School of Nursing at California State University, Chico, and past president of the Honor Society of Nursing, Sigma Theta Tau International.*

Unified Approach Needed for Entry to Practice

by Patrice K. Nicholas and Holly Fulmer

Among the most critical issues facing the nursing profession is the need to come to consensus on education for entry to practice. In the recent landmark report on nursing education, *Educating Nurses: A Call for Radical Transformation*, Benner and colleagues (2010) address the critical need to upgrade classroom education to prepare nurses for the complex clinical experiences that newly licensed nurses will encounter in clinical practice. In examining entry to practice and pathways, Benner et al. note that it is essential that the nursing profession require the BSN for entry to practice:

> *Unlike their colleague educators preparing lawyers, clergy, physicians, and engineers, nursing faculty and preceptors have relatively little time to build a*

discussion point

How would your day-to-day nursing practice change if each of your colleagues had a master's degree or other advanced degree?

Did you know …

The most commonly reported initial nursing education of RNs in the United States is the Associate Degree in Nursing (ADN), representing 45.4% of nurses. Bachelor's or graduate degrees were received by 34.2% of RNs, and 20.4% received their initial education in hospital-based diploma programs (USDHHS, 2010).

broad and deep knowledge base and guide students in professional formation. Yet nursing requires a high degree of responsibility and judgment in high-risk, underdetermined situations. Thus the baccalaureate degree in nursing should be the minimal educational level for entry into practice. . . . We challenge the profession to come to swift agreement about the most effective way to transform the current diverse pathways into a unified whole. (p. 216-217)

Further evidence of the importance of the baccalaureate degree in nursing comes from the recent Institute of Medicine report, *The Future of Nursing: Leading Change, Advancing Health*. In 2008, the Robert Wood Johnson Foundation and the Institute of Medicine launched this 2-year initiative to address the importance of transforming the nursing profession to meet the needs of our 21st century health care system. The report notes that varying levels of education and competencies impede effective care for patients and promoting health. Four key messages were delivered from this initiative:

- Nurses should practice to the full extent of their education and training.

- Nurses should achieve higher levels of education and training through an improved education system that promotes seamless academic progression.

- Nurses should be full partners, with physicians and other health care professionals, in redesigning health care in the United States.

- Effective workforce planning and policymaking require better data collection and an improved information infrastructure.

Although the report did not specifically address the BSN for entry to practice, the importance of nursing education and the attainment of competencies in leadership, health policy, system improvement, research and evidence-based practice, and teamwork and collaboration are viewed as essential. We suggest that these competencies can only be attained when there is agreement that the BSN should be the entry-to-practice approach to professional nursing education.

The 2010 Patient Protection and Affordable Care Act also requires that there be a National Health Care Workforce Commission to investigate the demand and preparation for the health professions. We write as a mentor and mentee who have experienced firsthand the importance of a baccalaureate-prepared education in the complex academic medical centers and technology-enhanced environments where professional nurses practice. The nursing profession is at the epicenter of profound changes in science, technology, and shifts in how and where care is provided. At no other time in history has it been as important that the baccalaureate degree be required for practice across the country and globally.

What do you think?

Did you know …

A national survey of deans and directors from U.S. nursing schools found that 65% of new BSN graduates had job offers at the time of graduation, which is substantially higher than the national average across all professions (24.4%). At 4 to 6 months after graduation, the survey found that 89% of new BSN graduates had secured job offers (American Association of Colleges of Nursing, 2010).

We also urge that the National Health Care Workforce Commission fully support the BSN as the entry-to-practice degree for professional nursing, just as the American Association of Colleges of Nursing, the American Nurses Association, and other leading nursing organizations have committed to in order to transform the current diverse pathways into a unified approach for entry to practice.

—**Patrice K. Nicholas,** *DNSc, RN, ANP, FAAN, is director of global health and academic partnerships at Brigham and Women's Hospital, professor at MGH Institute of Health Professions, and director for the Honor Society of Nursing, Sigma Theta Tau International.*

—**Holly Fulmer,** *BSN, RN, completed an advanced preceptor placement at Brigham and Women's Hospital (BWH) in Boston during her nursing education. She is a staff nurse on the gynecology oncology unit at BWH.*

"[We need to develop] consensus on entry into practice competencies and expectations at many levels, including now the advanced practice roles."

–**Karen Hill,** *DNP, RN, NEA-BC, vice president and nurse executive, Central Baptist Hospital, Lexington, Kentucky, USA*

Creating a Blueprint for the Future of Nursing

by Martha Dawson

The nursing profession has debated for more than 5 decades what should be the educational level for entry into nursing practice. Nurse leaders can best serve to strengthen the profession in this new era of opportunities by addressing and re-solving the entry into practice requirement. Moving to the Bachelor of Science in Nursing (BSN) degree as the required educational level for entry into practice is no longer an issue relating to just associate's degree (AD) prepared nurses.

Some 4-year nursing programs are granting students the right to take the NCLEX without awarding a degree; these programs are often designed to allow students to continue their education to the Master of Science in Nursing (MSN) or the Doctor of Nursing Practice (DNP) levels. Most AD nursing programs are operating with a "one plus two" educational curriculum, requiring 3 years for students to complete their AD program—1 year less than it takes to earn a BSN.

The need to transition the profession from multiple entry pathways to a single educational entry point (degree) is supported by a growing body of research and literature. There is evidence supporting the impact that BSN-prepared nurses have on length of stay, adverse events, and patient outcomes. The complexity of health care systems and the interprofessional aspect of nursing practice in all types

"Making the BSN the entry level for the profession [is important]. It still amazes me that we want to be considered 'professionals,' even with a two-year degree."

–**Cynthia Saver,** *MS, RN, president of CLS Development Inc., Columbia, Maryland, USA*

It's your turn ... start the discussion!

_____

_____

_____

_____

_____

_____

_____

_____

_____

_____

of settings require nurses who are educated to provide input into the planning of patient care, design of health care systems, and evaluation of care outcomes, and to contribute to the financial status of organizations as revenue generators.

"Minimum preparation of nursing—how low can we go? It is counterproductive to professional development because our basic credentials are not comparable with other health disciplines. Occupational therapists and physical therapists need master's degrees to practice, but we are using more and more health care aides to replace the shortage of nursing staffs."

–**Claudia Kam Yuk Lai**, *PhD, RN, professor, Hong Kong Polytechnic University School of Nursing, Hong Kong SAR, China*

The recent Robert Wood Johnson Foundation Report at the Institute of Medicine (2010) discussed the future of nursing and issued a call to action for nurse leaders and the profession.

The IOM report recommended an 80% BSN workforce by 2020 and a seamless education. If the profession continues to educate a significant number of its members at the AD level, it will be impossible to achieve the 80% BSN goal.

The IOM recommendation that community colleges evolve their AD nursing curricula into BSN programs must be given serious consideration by nursing education accrediting bodies, and by deans and policymakers at the state level. Transitioning community colleges' AD programs to BSN curricula will allow university-based schools of nursing to shift their focus to preparing more master's and DNP graduates to meet the growing needs for nursing faculty, advanced practitioners, and nursing scientists.

Nurse leaders, boards of nursing, policymakers, and college and university presidents should begin dialogue to promote nursing as a science-based profession that requires the BSN as the pre-licensure education level. The current economic environment and the need for more nurses cannot support the current multiple routes of nursing education that extend cost. Nurse leaders should unite and create a blueprint to move the profession into the future and declare the BSN as the minimum educational level for entry into practice in the United States.

—**Martha A. Dawson**, *DNP, MSN, FACHE, is chief executive officer of MA Dawson & Associates and assistant professor at the University of Alabama at Birmingham.*

"Further advancement of minimum of nursing education [is needed], i.e., BSN."

–**Vicki Michelle McMahon**, MSN, RN

References

American Association of Colleges of Nursing. (2010, November 10). *AACN data confirm that nurses with bachelor's degrees are more likely to secure jobs sooner after graduation than other professionals*. Retrieved from http://www.aacn.nche.edu/media/newsreleases/2010/bsngrad.html

Benner, P., Sutphen, M., Leonard, V., & Day, L. (2010). *Educating nurses: A call for radical transformation*. Stanford, CA: Carnegie Foundation for the Advancement of Nursing/Jossey Bass.

Institute of Medicine. (2011). *The future of nursing. Leading change, advancing health*. Washington, DC: The National Academies Press.

Robert Wood Johnson Foundation Initiative on the Future of Nursing at the Institute of Medicine. (2010). *The future of nursing: Leading change, advancing health*. Washington, DC: Institute of Medicine.

U.S. Department of Health and Human Services (USDHHS). (2010). *The registered nurse population: Findings from the 2008 National Sample Survey of Registered Nurses*. Retrieved from http://www.thefutureof-nursing.org/sites/default/files/RN%20Nurse%20Population.pdf

Question #4:

Nursing Education Part II: DNP vs. PhD— Separate but Equal?

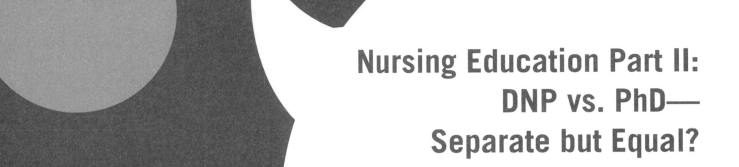

Did you know ...

As reported in April 2011, 153 DNP programs are currently enrolling students at schools of nursing nationwide, and an additional 160 DNP programs are in the planning stages (American Association of Colleges of Nursing, 2011).

Want to open a can of worms at a nursing education conference? Bring up the PhD versus DNP debate! When the Doctor of Nursing Practice (DNP) was introduced in 2004, a lot of arguments erupted over why it was a bad idea. The naysayers threatened to sink it before the first graduates even collected their diplomas.

Fortunately, within a few short years, the degree has stabilized and is even starting to catch on, offering a practical option to many nurses looking for a clinical alternative to a research-focused doctorate. However, the fact remains: There is a lot of resistance to the idea of an alternate terminal degree for nurses—one that isn't grounded in academic research. The issue? Academics and researchers perceive that an advanced practice nursing degree must be easier to complete than a traditional PhD, grounded in academic research. I mean, who wouldn't want to be out in the clinical setting instead of behind all those library stacks? But when you look at the curriculum of most DNP programs, the academic rigor is present. The degrees are different, but as terminal degrees go, they are equally difficult.

So what will it take for us to have a rational discussion about both of these degrees? Sure, there are a lot of additional questions that concern everyone, such as faculty tenure, but can we at least agree that they are separate but equal?

Other health care professions, such as pharmacology and speech/language pathology, have comparable doctorate-level degrees of practice. Why not agree that nursing isn't so different and that two terminal degrees—both requiring the same amount of work—give nurses the opportunity to pursue what will truly make them better nurses? Decisions can't be reached until we start the conversation.

Can We Double the Number of Doctorally Prepared Nurses?

by Geraldine Bednash

The release of the Institute of Medicine (IOM) report *The Future of Nursing: Leading Change, Advancing Health* (2011) provides the nursing profession with specific challenges that must be addressed to ensure that we fulfill our social responsibility to provide high-quality, patient-centered, and safe health care.

One notable recommendation was the validation of the need for a marked enhancement in the educational preparation of professional nurses from the beginning baccalaureate degree to the terminal doctoral degree. The IOM Commission called for an increase in the percentage of professional nurses who hold the baccalaureate degree to 80% by 2020 and for a doubling of nurses who are doctorally educated. These goals were established in direct response to the growing base of evidence documenting the impact of a better educated nursing workforce on care quality and safety.

Another of the report's goals is to prepare doctorally educated nurses who will shape advanced clinical practice, supply the evidence for all nursing practice, and serve as the future professionals who will provide expert nursing care. The IOM Committee's recommendation to double the number of nurses with doctorates was focused on expansion of graduates from both the Doctor of Philosophy (PhD) research-focused programs and the Doctor of Nursing Practice (DNP) clinical practice programs.

discussion point

If you were going to pursue a graduate degree in nursing, would you pursue a DNP or a PhD? Why or why not?

Did you know …

DNP programs are now available in 37 states plus the District of Columbia. States with the most programs (more than five) include Florida, Illinois, Massachusetts, Minnesota, New York, Ohio, Pennsylvania, and Texas.

(American Association of Colleges of Nursing, 2011)

Expanding the population of doctorally prepared nurses must be accompanied by a major culture change in nursing that encourages new entrants into the profession to move rapidly through graduate education. This cultural change will encounter some resistance from individuals who hold outdated notions of career development. Nursing leaders and other stakeholders must evolve their thinking and understand the importance of this shift. The historical pattern of encouraging new graduates to enter the workforce for several years prior to graduate education has created multiple barriers to efforts focused on expanding the educational preparation of our professional workforce and has elongated significantly the trajectory to the terminal degree.

Recent decisions by the nursing profession to change the requirement for preparation at the highest level of practice from the master's degree to the DNP must be accompanied by efforts to recruit new graduates to these programs.

Additionally, the need to expand the cadre of nurses who seek careers as scientists must be addressed through systematic and organized efforts to mentor future research-focused doctoral students early in their professional formation as part of their entry-level baccalaureate degree programs.

Over the last decade, our nation has seen dramatic calls for change in the education of all health professionals, not just nurses. Nurses must take a proactive approach to ensuring that we are preparing a future workforce that can address these calls for change and adapt to a new dynamic in care delivery.

The continuing evolution and expansion of the science framing expert clinical care challenge educators of all health professions in their efforts to shape curriculum. Nursing is responding with the decision to move to the DNP for the preparation of advanced practice registered nurses and through other efforts, such as the clinical nurse leader initiative. Clinical practice is now shaped by not just the science of clinical interventions but also by the science of genetics, informatics, and economics. A commitment to enhancing the educational preparation of nurses must be accompanied by a commitment to moving ahead rapidly to shape a professional culture that encourages and rewards progressive academic achievement.

—**Geraldine Bednash**, *PhD, RN, FAAN, is chief executive officer and executive director, American Association of Colleges of Nursing.*

Top 10 challenges

"[There is an] increasing drive to raise academic standards in nurse education—the United Kingdom is moving to an all-degree profession."

—**Matthew Aldridge**, BSc (Hons) Clinical Nursing Practice, MA (Ed), RN, Registered Nurse Teacher, FHEA, senior lecturer in acute adult nursing, University of Wolverhampton

Changing Health Care Environment Calls for More Highly Educated Nurses

by Karen Profitt Newman

In May 2010, the Tri-Council for Nursing issued a consensus position statement on the Educational Advancement of Registered Nurses. Subsequently, in October 2010, the Institute of Medicine (IOM) and the Robert Wood Johnson Foundation (RWJF) released *The Future of Nursing: Leading Change, Advancing Health* (IOM, 2011), with recommendations for action that include higher levels of education and training through an improved education system that promotes seamless academic progression.

Both of these timely documents address the prominent role of nurses in transforming the U.S. health care system in response to the sweeping legislation of the 2010 Patient Protection and Affordable Care Act. These two reports follow closely the introduction by the American Association of Colleges of Nursing (AACN) in 2007 of the clinical nurse leader (CNL) role, and the AACN position statement (2004) on the practice doctorate in nursing (DNP).

Clearly, the health care system is rapidly evolving, and the health care environment—including technology, medical therapies, and treatments—is increasingly complex. These factors, along with the predicted nursing shortage and impending tsunami of aging baby boomers who "will not go gently into that good night" of retirement and declining health, all combine to underscore the need not only for *more* registered nurses but more *highly educated* nurses.

To apply Malcolm Gladwell's phrase, it would appear that we are at a tipping point in society as it relates to our health care system and in the nursing profession, since the 3 million nurses in this country represent the nation's largest workforce.

I believe some of the major challenges for nursing education at this pivotal time include the following:

- Streamlining educational progression to facilitate increasing numbers of advanced practice nurses

- Actionable collaboration among nursing education, practice, and professional associations to promote academic progression

- Clear role definition and articulation of the value amid the "alphabet soup" of advanced practice nurses (CNS, CNL, ARNP, APRN, DNP, CRNA, CNM, DNSc, DNS, PhD)

- Increased funding for advanced nursing education in this economic climate

- Removal of barriers to practice and reimbursement for advanced practice nurses

discussion point

In your current organization, would there be any benefit for you to obtain an advanced nursing degree? Which one? Why?

Did you know …

From 2009 to 2010, the number of students enrolled in DNP programs increased from 5,165 to 7,034. During that same period, the number of DNP graduates nearly doubled: from 660 to 1,282. (American Association of Colleges of Nursing, 2011)

All of these challenges require committed, engaged nursing leaders who are competent in communication and relationship-building, are knowledgeable of the rapidly changing health care environment, and possess leadership, professionalism, business skills, and political influence.

—**Karen Profitt Newman**, *EdD, MSN, RN, NEA-BC, is vice president and chief nursing officer at Baptist Hospital East in Louisville, Kentucky, USA.*

The DNP: Key to Standardizing Advanced Practice Nursing Education?

by Kristene Diggins

When contemplating the future role of the Doctor of Nursing Practice (DNP) degree, we must consider the history of advanced practice nursing. According to the widely used Internet encyclopedia Wikipedia (2011, January), an advanced practice nurse (APN) is "a registered nurse who has completed specific advanced nursing education and training in the diagnosis and management of common, as well as a few complex, medical conditions. APNs are generally licensed through nursing boards rather than medical boards. They provide a broad range of health care services."

This definition falls short. Even the regulatory definition of NP practice varies from state to state. For example, in North Carolina, where I practice, NPs are regulated by a joint commission of the medical and nursing boards. Trying to find a standard definition is made even more difficult by the lack of a regulatory standard in the health care industry itself.

As we consider the vast array in scopes of practice and nursing education for APNs, the DNP degree could provide the standardization we are pursuing. During the past 35 years, the NP role has expanded throughout the country. The scope of practice for NPs varies from state to state, and throughout the country, there is an increasing need for the services NPs provide. So, standardizing APN training is at the forefront of the needs of health care.

Leaders in the nursing profession have tried to address this need with the DNP. This is an innovative way for APNs to meet the expanding knowledge demands of providing health care today. And yet, we know that the nursing shortage limits the availability of faculty and students. For this very reason, the National Council of State Boards of Nursing recently met to discuss its position on APN practice, which is to embrace a unified approach to regulation of APN practice.

Once again, nursing is at a crossroads where demand for nurses and standardization of APN training could determine the future of educational goals. It is important to provide a degree that standardizes APN training and, in so doing, provides a unified approach to advance practice nursing. This will hopefully attract more nursing students to nursing and promote the APN role nationwide.

discussion point

Does the "alphabet soup" of nurse credentials, including advanced degrees, help or harm nursing's (and nurses') reputation among other professional groups? How so?

Did you know …

Beginning in 2015, the American Association of Colleges of Nursing will require all entry-level nurse practitioner programs (including clinical nurse specialists and nurse midwives) to transition from the MSN degree to the DNP degree. In addition, by the year 2025, the American Association of Nurse Anesthetists will require the DNP degree for entry-level nurse anesthetist programs. However, nurse practitioners and nurse anesthetists in practice prior to those dates will not be required to have the DNP degree (Marshall, 2010).

As we can deduce from the NCSBN APRN consensus model, by 2015 there will be a unified approach to both the education and practice of APNs nationwide. This will empower APNs to further advance their pivotal role in health care today.

—**Kristene Diggins**, *DNP, RN, is a certified nurse practitioner in geriatrics and family practice, working with Wycliffe Bible Translators at a mission clinic as well as at a health clinic for the elderly. She teaches online for the University of Phoenix/Axia College.*

Putting the Essentials of Doctoral Education Into Practice

by Kimberly Adams Tufts

The nursing profession is at the proverbial crossroads. Of late, there have been calls for a more highly educated (Institute of Medicine, 2011) and a differently educated nursing workforce (Benner, Sutphen, Leonard, & Day, 2010). A world where emerging technology and advanced diagnostics contribute to the ever-growing complexity of health care delivery, where changing demography has resulted in a newly emerging sociocultural majority with a diversity of health care needs, and where professional standards are based not on where we are in nursing but where we want to go provides us with a window of opportunity for transforming nurse education in fundamental ways.

Benner and colleagues (2010) state that a considerable gap exists between the current nursing practice environment and nursing education. The emergence of the

Doctor of Nursing Practice (DNP) educational programs portends to be one solution to our changing practice environment. The history of DNP education is short albeit significant. In October 2004, the member schools of the American Association of Colleges of Nursing (AACN) voted to endorse the position statement on the practice doctorate in nursing, calling for educational preparation for advanced nursing practice to move from the master's to the doctoral level by 2015.

AACN then moved forth to publish *The Essentials of Doctoral Education for Advanced Nursing Practice* (2006). This document outlines eight requisite competencies that must guide the development of advanced practice curricula:

1. Scientific foundations for practice

2. Organizational and systems leadership

3. Clinical scholarship

4. Information systems/technology

5. Health policy

6. Interprofessional collaboration

7. Clinical prevention and population health

8. Advanced nursing practice

Adherence to the principles embodied in the *Essentials* document is essential to the successful transformation of advanced practice education, ultimately

discussion point

Should only faculty members with a PhD, DNS, or EdD teach nursing students? Why or why not? Can you imagine a scenario where a DNP might be the more qualified instructor? Why or why not?

It's your turn ... start the discussion!

_____

_____

_____

_____

_____

_____

_____

_____

_____

_____

_____

_____

improving nursing practice and resulting in more optimal population health outcomes. Adhering to these principles will provide nurse educators with building blocks for educating nurses who are prepared to impact health care delivery to vulnerable populations from diverse backgrounds who have a variety of health needs, whether centered around pregnancy prenatal care for childbearing women, obesity prevention and interventions for school-aged children, risk reduction for minority populations, self-management skills for persons living with HIV, health literacy programming for the elderly, providing mobile health services to rural bound-persons, or other needs.

Providing a nursing education that puts the _Essentials_ at the core of DNP education has the potential to increase knowledge, to change attitudes, and to facilitate the acquisition of new skills. Yet it will not be enough to "cover" the _Essentials_. An education that revolves around the _Essentials_ must provide opportunities to apply the competencies to the practice environment—to use them as a framework for trialing new ideas, as a guide for structured reflection, and as the template for translating research into practice.

Nurses who are on the receiving end of such an education will be positioned to sit at the table, substantially contributing to public policy conversations, assuming leadership positions, and—most importantly—transforming nursing practice as well as patient outcomes (Olshanky, 2004).

—**Kimberly Adams Tufts**, _DNP, WHNP-BC, FAAN, is associate professor and director of community and global initiatives at Old Dominion University in Norfolk, Virginia, USA._

References

American Association of Colleges of Nursing. (2004, October). *AACN position statement on the practice doctorate in nursing*. Retrieved from http://www.aacn.nche.edu/dnp/dnppositionstatement.htm

American Association of Colleges of Nursing. (2006). *The essentials of doctoral education for advanced nursing practice*. Retrieved from http://www.aacn.nche.edu/DNP/pdf/Essentials.pdf

American Association of Colleges of Nursing. (2007). *White paper on the role of the clinical nurse leader*. Retrieved from http://www.aacn.nche.edu/Publications/WhitePapers/ClinicalNurseLeader.htm

American Association of Colleges of Nursing. (2011, April). *The Doctor of Nursing Practice (DNP)*. Retrieved from http://www.aacn.nche.edu/media/FactSheets/dnp.htm

Benner, P., Sutphen, M., Leonard, V., & Day, L. (2010). *Educating nurses: A call for radical transformation*. San Francisco: Jossey-Bass.

Institute of Medicine. (2011). *The future of nursing. Leading change, advancing health*. Washington, DC: The National Academies Press.

Institute of Medicine. (2010). *The future of nursing: focus on education*. Retrieved from http://www.iom.edu/~/media/Files/Report%20Files/2010/The-Future-of-Nursing/Nursing%20Education%202010%20Brief.pdf

Marshall, L. (2010). *Take charge of your nursing career*. Indianapolis, IN: Sigma Theta Tau International.

Olshansky, E. (2004). Are nurses at the table? A new nursing degree could help. *Journal of Professional Nursing*, *20*(4), 211-212.

Wikipedia. (2011, January). *Advanced practice nurse*. Retrieved from http://en.wikipedia.org/wiki/Advanced_practice_nurse

Notes

Question #5:

How Do Nurses Get a Seat at the Policy Table?

discussion point

Every aspect of a nurse's practice is regulated by policy. What are three policy rules or regulations from your organization or state that you'd lobby to change for nursing?

_____

_____

_____

_____

_____

_____

It's such a difficult question. Nurses are caregivers, not politicians. For goodness sake, most of you warn each other, "Don't volunteer for that committee or task force—it will bleed you dry! The conflict! The endless debate! Don't do it!"

We know you've heard it. You've probably lived it. But if nurses want to be real players in shaping the future of their profession, they are going to have to step up and take that seat at the table—demand it, even! Nurses need to put aside the differences that divided them in the past and speak with a unified, professional, confident voice. Whether it's an organizational group or a professional opportunity, they need to put aside their timidity and insist that their voices be heard.

"But," you say, "I already volunteer for those committees. I sit in on those meetings. I don't shy away from being considered a nurse leader, and nurses are not heard. The problem is that half the time, we don't even get a seat! So how do nurses get there?"

Nurses need to work together. They need to find one voice. They need to be skilled advocates for themselves, their patients, and their profession. Nurses have to be aware of policy. They must be aware of their representation in leadership positions of their organizations and universities at every level, from the bedside to the boardroom.

Nurses need to have a say. But instead of waiting to be asked, they need to step up and take their seat. Part of being a qualified caregiver is using your voice to advocate for your patients. Let's start a conversation about how you can advocate for yourselves.

Top 10 challenges

"All of the national agendas for health care reform will impact either the advancement of nursing or the limitation of nursing. Nursing's leadership is essential, not as a fight for power but the assurance that the voice and wisdom of the largest health care group of professionals who are present at the point of care—the place where the hands of those who give and receive care meet—help create a transformed health care system."

—Bonnie Wesorick, MSN, RN, FAAN, founder of CPM Resource Center, Grand Rapids, Michigan, USA

What do you think?

_____

_____

_____

_____

_____

_____

_____

_____

_____

_____

_____

Did you know ...

From *The Future of Nursing: Leading Change, Advancing Health* (Institute of Medicine, 2011):

> Traditional nursing competencies such as case management and coordination, patient education, public health intervention, and transitional care are likely to dominate in a reformed health care system as it inevitably moves toward an emphasis on prevention and management rather than acute care (O'Neil, 2009).

Once-in-a-Lifetime Opportunities for Nurses, From the Bedside to the Boardroom

by Karen A. Daley

As our nation undertakes transformative health care reform, nurses have unprecedented opportunities to optimize their practice, drive change, and shape the health care system of the future. Imagine how patients and communities would benefit if all 3 million nurses practiced to the full extent of their knowledge, skills, and education. Imagine the impact you could make in countless lives and how your professional competence and satisfaction would grow.

Both the new health care law, the Affordable Care Act (ACA), and the Institute of Medicine's report on the future of nursing call for a larger role for nurses in providing patient-centered care in a reformed health care system.

It is an exciting time for the profession, and each and every nurse—from the bedside to the boardroom—has a role to play in the many stages of reform. Nurses' knowledge and expertise are in demand, and how we rise to meet today's challenges will influence how our health care system looks in 10 years.

The American Nurses Association has advocated for comprehensive reform for decades, and we support full implementation of the ACA. It is a comprehensive law that aims to protect consumers, increase access to care, promote health, improve and refocus the health care delivery system, and control costs. The law creates wider opportunities for nurses to play a larger role in the delivery of care and supports development of a strong nursing workforce.

It includes such "nursing care" reforms as a greater emphasis on quality improvement: reporting, including nursing-sensitive measures; funding for a range of new innovative nursing education programs; and funding for nurse-managed health centers and other nurse-led models of care. These are among the changes that will help transform our system from one focused largely on "sick care" to one focused on health promotion, disease prevention, and care coordination.

Of course, much work remains to be done. Nurses must use their voices to oppose efforts to repeal, weaken, or deny funding for critical reforms within the current law. Rules and regulations are still being developed, and implementation will ultimately occur at the state, local, and community levels. We need to remain steadfast in our commitment to health care reform and engage in the policy development process within the political arena. We must seize this once-in-a-lifetime opportunity and use our trusted voice to ensure that we achieve the vision of a patient-centered, quality-driven health care system.

—**Karen A. Daley**, *PhD, MPH, RN, FAAN, is president of the American Nurses Association.*

Top 10 challenges

"The challenge for the profession is to be engaged, involved, and respected, as well as invited to the policymaking tables."

—**Daniel J. Pesut**, PhD, RN, PMHCNS-BC, FAAN, professor, Indiana University School of Nursing, Indianapolis, Indiana, USA

Top 10 challenges

"Despite all the effort to get a seat at the table, it still seems like doctors get all the attention and nurses get left behind. The good news has been NPs getting noticed because of health care reform. But still, much more needs to be done."

—**Cynthia Saver**, MS, RN, president of CLS Development, Inc.

Did you know ...

Hospitals remain the most common employment setting for RNs in the United States, increasing from 57.4% in 2004 to 62.2% of employed RNs in 2008. The increase in this percentage is the first increase since 1984 (U.S. Department of Health and Human Services, 2010).

Nurses As Health Care and Workforce Reform Agents

by Tine Hansen-Turton

An inadequate U.S. health care workforce is the Achilles' heel of President Obama's health care reform law. In the face of acute primary care physician shortages and steady reductions in the number of physicians who are willing to accept government programs, our existing primary care system will not be able to meet the needs of the approximately 32 million Americans who soon will become insured through national health care reform. Furthermore, health care delivery is strained under tremendous pressure from the demands of chronic health diseases. So what needs to happen to make health care reform a success? The answer is simple: Look to nursing in solving this impending workforce disaster. Nurses have been part of the solution for 5 decades. We just haven't paid attention to them as a nation.

In recent years, there have been a series of "disruptive innovations," a term coined by Harvard Professor Clayton Christensen, in the health care sector. One example of such an innovation is the growing movement of nurses—including nurse practitioners—providing high-quality primary and preventive care in retail-based settings and in community settings such as nurse-managed health clinics (NMHCs). Research by Deloitte Health Solutions and RAND Corporation and recent publications in *Health Affairs*, along with the Institute of Medicine (2011) report, *The Future of Nursing, Leading Change, Advancing Health*, have documented that these nurse-led clinics and other innovations provide safe, accessible, affordable care to millions of Americans and can be expanded. Patients gravitate to nurse-led care. For health care reform to be successful, just like patients who vote with their feet, we need to embrace these and many other "disruptive innovations."

So what's the lesson for nursing? Disruptive innovation does not happen overnight or without a strategy. It is built on a series of innovations that happen over time and usually grow and mature outside the limelight. Neither the retail clinics nor nurse-run clinics would exist without NPs in the primary care service seat. The NP workforce, today making up more than 150,000 with an annual growth rate of 5,500, was first established more than 50 years ago as a response to health care reform needs at that time—namely, a physician shortage and a belief that nursing could play a critical role in primary care.

It grew slowly, focused on taking care of people who needed access to care and, over time, gained patient trust and ultimately public support. Nursing has always been part of health care reform, but it has done so outside the limelight with a focus toward the solution of broadening the workforce. It is time for nursing to stand up and claim its value as the true health care and workforce reform agent in the U.S.

–**Tine Hansen-Turton**, *MGA, JD, is vice president of health care access and policy at Public Health Management Corporation and CEO of the National Nursing Centers Consortium.*

discussion point

Do you feel like your interests parallel the nursing profession's interests? Is what you think is best for the patient also best for the profession? For you? (Don't worry. There are no "right" answers here.)

Did you know ...

What's important:

"To ensure that all Americans have access to needed health care services and that nurses' unique contributions to the health care team are maximized, federal and state actions are required to update and standardize scope of practice regulations to take advantage of the full capacity of education of APRNs" (Institute of Medicine, 2011).

We Have the Blueprint: Let's Work Together to Improve Patient Care!

by Susan B. Hassmiller

Health reform discussions often center on expanding access to care, improving health care quality, and controlling health care costs. Policymakers wrestle with caring for an aging population, managing more patients with chronic conditions, improving care coordination, addressing health care disparities, and providing end-of-life care. Nurses can—and indeed must—fill many of these roles. As the largest segment of the health care workforce and the health professionals who spend the most time with patients, nurses have a vital role to play in transforming our health care system.

In October 2010, the Institute of Medicine (IOM) released a landmark report called *The Future of Nursing: Leading Change, Advancing Health* (Institute of Medicine, 2011) that calls for improvements in public and institutional policies at the national, state, and local levels to transform nursing to improve patient care. The recommendations seek to expand opportunities for nurses to lead, expand scope of practice, improve education, and enhance data collection.

The Robert Wood Johnson Foundation (RWJF) believes that these recommendations, if implemented, would result in wide-reaching improvements in the health care system and directly improve patient care. In November 2010, RWJF launched *The Future of Nursing: Campaign for Action* to advance the IOM recommendations. RWJF is collaborating with AARP to organize a nonpartisan coalition dedicated to advancing the IOM recommendations. Partners include health professionals, payers, consumers, business leaders, policymakers, philanthropies, educators, hospitals and health systems, and public health agencies. Addressing nursing workforce challenges must be considered a societal issue that belongs to all who consider health care a priority.

RWJF and AARP are developing Regional Action Coalitions (RACs) that will move key nursing-related issues forward at the local, state, and national levels. We are working with groups in 15 states and will later move nationwide. It is vital for all nurses to join an RAC. Leadership begins at every level: from the bedside to the boardroom. We can't rely only on senior nursing leaders to reform the nation's health care system. Everyone must be involved. RACs are recruiting stakeholders from a variety of sectors; educating policymakers and other decision-makers on issues; reaching out to philanthropies to seek financial support; engaging the media; and moving key recommendations forward. Sign up at www.thefutureofnursing.org.

We have an opportunity to transform nursing in order to improve patient care. The IOM has laid out an action-oriented blueprint; the nursing leadership is united and other partners have joined us. Let's work together to make wide-reaching improvements to directly improve patient care.

—**Susan B. Hassmiller**, *PhD, RN, FAAN, is senior adviser for nursing at the Robert Wood Johnson Foundation and director, Robert Wood Johnson Initiative on the Future of Nursing, at the Institute of Medicine.*

It's your turn... start the discussion!

References

Institute of Medicine. (2011). *The future of nursing. Leading change, advancing health*. Washington, DC: The National Academies Press.

O'Neil, E. (2009). Four factors that guarantee health care change. *Journal of Professional Nursing, 25*(6), 317-321.

U.S. Department of Health and Human Services (USDHHS). (2010). *The registered nurse population: Findings from the 2008 National Sample Survey of Registered Nurses*. Retrieved from http://www.thefutureof-nursing.org/sites/default/files/RN%20Nurse%20Population.pdf

Question #6:

How Do Nurses Cope With the Growing Ethical Demands of Practice?

discussion point

Given the first scenario mentioned in this chapter—the preemie versus the elderly man—make a decision based on your position as a staff nurse caring for the gentleman. Now make a decision as the nurse manager whose performance is evaluated on managing costs and patient beds. What about as the CEO of the hospital, who is responsible for hundreds of jobs?

_____
_____
_____
_____
_____

When it comes to ethics in nursing, you can encounter the proverbial sticky wickets everywhere you look. Is removing life-sustaining technology from a 24-week-old preemie with numerous complications and little chance of surviving more difficult than removing it from an 80-year-old man with COPD and pneumonia whose lungs will never function on their own again? Both patients are consuming thousands of dollars' worth of care—and countless employee hours—with doubtful benefit. But the families of both patients are distraught and unwilling to "pull the plug."

The preemie's parents want everything medically possible done to save their baby's life. They say they've heard about health care rationing and want no part of it. The children of the elderly patient say he had a good quality of life until he developed pneumonia; they think the hospital wants him to die because his care is costing too much money, a situation similar to the "death panels" they've heard about.

How do nurses help their patients' families sort through their highly charged emotions and explain the difference between futility and possibility and the inexact science of modern medicine? The often unanswerable ethical situations that abound in the 21st century already cause enough moral distress among health care professionals.

Unfortunately, recent political rhetoric, half-truths, outright lies, and biased media reports continue to do a disservice to both the American public and health care providers, especially when it comes to end-of-life care.

Nurses can head off the damage done by this misinformation by talking to their own families and friends and their patients before they have to deal with end-of-life concerns. If you don't ask Grandma if she wants a G-tube or ventilator, who will?

Nursing organizations, associations, and leaders need to step out of the shadows and educate themselves and their patients. It's time to lead the discussion instead of just listening.

What do you think?

Did you know ...

Ethics for nurses permeate every aspect of practice, not just end-of-life or palliative care. Ethical issues can include patient communication, professionalism in the workplace, cultural dilemmas, and even migration issues as more nurses work in different workplace and cultural environments.

Nurses: Add Your Voice to Discussion on Ethics

by Connie M. Ulrich

The nursing profession faces significant ethical challenges in meeting the future demands of patients within their care. The health statistics of the nation are astounding in terms of an increasingly aging and chronically ill population; in fact, by 2030, the number of older persons in the United States will almost double, and those age 65 and older will represent 19%—nearly one fifth—of the population (U.S. Census Bureau, 2010).

Difficult ethical questions arise as older adults suffer the burden of many chronic diseases, such as cancer, Alzheimer's disease, diabetes, heart disease, and many other physiological and neurological insults. Additionally, our ability to use emerging technological and genetic information to assist patients and their families in determining what is in their best interest can carry weighty moral concerns.

Nurses are front-line providers of care in our society and are a highly trusted professional group. However, they continue to confront daily ethical concerns about how to protect patients' rights and address issues of informed consent, end-of-life questions, allocation of scarce resources, and surrogate decision-making, among other problems, within institutionalized health care settings. As such, they are increasingly distressed and dissatisfied, and express feelings of powerlessness to effect change. Nurses often struggle with knowing how to help patients make dignified choices when they might believe that the choice that was made only prolonged human suffering and perhaps was neither the best, nor most dignified, choice.

How do nurses care *for* and care *about* patients in environments that are "fast-paced" and "ethically loaded," and sometimes reflect "bottom-line" profit practices? Today, the phenomenon of *moral distress* (knowing the morally correct action but being unable to act on it because of various internal or external constraints) is a common occurrence in nursing practice. Indeed, about one out of four nurses reports he or she will leave the profession because of moral distress (Ulrich et al., 2007).

With a looming nursing shortage, serious attention to the ethical demands of caregiving in the workplace is needed. Simply ignoring or failing to address ethics-related problems in the delivery of nursing care will not diminish its pervasive impact. We must create a climate of mutual respect among physicians and nurses working within health care institutions, so both groups of providers can equally contribute to the dialogue on quality patient care.

Nurses need to feel empowered to use their voices for the patient's good and to do so with confidence. This type of dialogue can begin in the classroom. *The Future*

discussion point

Do you fear losing your job if you go against a physician's or the institution's policies in order to do the right thing, such as refusing to administer meds you know to be erroneous for a patient? If yes, what would have to change to make you feel safe as an ethical patient advocate?

Top 10
challenges

"[One of the top challenges
facing the profession is] nurses'
understanding and use of genetics
information in the counseling, care,
and treatment of certain diseases,
as well as the ethical issues related
to consumer access, understanding,
and consequences of genetic
engineering and use."

–**Daniel J. Pesut**, PhD, RN,
PMHCNS-BC, FAAN, professor,
Indiana University School of Nursing,
Indianapolis, Indiana, USA

of Nursing: Leading Change, Advancing Health (Institute of Medicine, 2011) calls for innovative training-related reforms to prepare nurses for the upcoming challenges they will undoubtedly face. Interdisciplinary ethics education should be part of that call.

—**Connie M. Ulrich**, *PhD, RN, FAAN, is associate professor of nursing and bioethics at the University of Pennsylvania School of Nursing and a senior fellow at the Center for Bioethics. She holds a secondary appointment with the School of Medicine in the Department of Medical Ethics.*

Nurses Face Increased Ethical Demands and Moral Distress

by Karen H. Morin

Advances in technology, an aging population, societal pressure to control health care costs and to reform health care, increasing numbers of chronically ill people, and the presence of health disparities increase the number of multifaceted ethical issues nurses are called on to address (Robinson, 2010; Ulrich & Hamric, 2008). Frequently, ethical issues arise in relation to pain management, quality of life, resource allocations, and end-of-life (Dierkx de Casterlé, Izumi, Godfrey, & Denhaerynck, 2008; Kain, 2007; Olmstead, Scott, & Austin, 2010). In confronting these issues, nurses may experience moral distress.

What is moral distress? McCarthy and Deady (2008) indicate that people experience moral distress when they "make moral judgements about the right course of action to take in a situation, and they are unable to carry it out" (p. 254). To this, the American Association of Critical-Care Nurses (2006) adds situations in which actions are demanded that are contrary to a nurse's personal and professional values.

What are the consequences of moral distress? A review of research findings reveals that experiencing moral distress exerts a personal toll on nurses, has the potential to impact patient care, and can negatively affect organizational functioning (Corley, 2002; McCarthy & Deady, 2008; Robinson, 2010). Investigators have found that nurses may experience self-doubt, disappointment, and even compromised personal integrity. Often, nurses respond to such experiences by leaving the offending place of employment, thus contributing to organizational recruitment and retention issues. Although negative effects of moral distress have been reported extensively, some investigators have identified strategies nurses employ to counteract these effects (McCarthy & Deady, 2008).

What challenges exist? One critical challenge relates to the definition of moral distress. McCarthy and Deady (2008) assert that much of the research literature lacks conceptual clarity. They question whether moral distress is a situation, a group of symptoms, or a range of emotions and, as an alternative, suggest it may be better conceptualized as a cluster concept, with the caveat that "understanding moral distress as a cluster concept should prompt caution in its description and use" (p. 259). Nurse scientists will need to address this challenge.

discussion point

Identify three ethical issues you have encountered in your workplace in the past 2 months that were not life-or-death issues, but presented a situation where you had to consider the right thing to do within ethical boundaries.

discussion point

What's the most difficult moral dilemma you've ever faced? How did you resolve it? Do you and your colleagues discuss moral dilemmas to compare notes and offer each other support?

_____

_____

_____

_____

_____

_____

Given the need for a diverse workforce, another challenge is to identify cultural influences that affect ethical decision-making and moral distress. Caldwell, Lu, and Harding (2010) advocate for increased attention to the use of multiple moral paradigms that are based on diverse cultural traditions.

A third challenge is to provide avenues by which health care professionals can discuss ethical issues without constraint. Ulrich and Hamric (2008) suggest implementing preventive ethics as one approach. Ramsey and colleagues (2010) identify a novel approach to enhance discussion of ethical issues: a secure (encrypted and password-protected) online ethics forum that "incorporates a priority system to alert members of pressing patient situations" (p. 16). Wocial et al. (2010) provide evidence supporting the use of unit-based ethics conversations. These strategies acknowledge the critical role enhanced communication plays in addressing and alleviating moral distress.

Finally, nurses are challenged to contribute to ethics-related discussions. Wright and Brajtman (2011) suggest that the integration of relational and embodied ethics knowledge enables nurses to bring a unique moral perspective to these discussions. As is evident from the preceding, there are multiple opportunities for nurses to exercise creativity in addressing moral distress. Key to success in addressing these challenges is inclusion of staff nurses, as well as colleagues from other disciplines.

—**Karen H. Morin**, *DSN, RN, ANEF, is the 2009-11 president of the Honor Society of Nursing, Sigma Theta Tau International and professor and director of the PhD program at the University of Wisconsin-Milwaukee.*

Ethical Dilemmas Heightened in End-of-Life Care

by Katherine Brown-Saltzman

A 5-year literature search using the key words "nursing" and "ethics" in 1985 retrieved 1,320 articles; a search covering the past 5 years revealed an astounding 4,435 articles—more than triple the 1985 number. Studies on "moral distress" during those same time periods climbed a staggering 1,900%: from nine to 174. This increase reflects what we are seeing in clinical practice and ethics consultation: ethical issues are growing in volume and complexity.

Perhaps the top ethical issues relate to end-of-life care, where the challenges are heightened and moral distress is often the greatest. Technology continues to proliferate and find its way into the mainstream as more Americans die in hospitals with aggressive treatments.

The statistics demonstrate that it is the last 2 years of life that consume the greatest portion of Medicare's budget. Last year, $30 billion was spent on non-beneficial end-of-life treatment. In between all those numbers are patients and families struggling to make difficult choices. These decisions are based largely upon a radical shift in health care over the last 30 years that has made patient autonomy a priority. Patients and families are now routinely asked what they want for treatment, often without regard to what is medically appropriate, let alone best

What do you think?

_____

_____

_____

_____

_____

_____

_____

_____

_____

_____

_____

_____

_____

discussion point

When's the last time you read your institution's code of ethics? If it's been awhile, read it. Did anything surprise you? What? Why? Would you change anything? What? Why?

_____

_____

_____

_____

_____

_____

from the perspective of overall wellness and health. Harmful treatments are routinely provided despite impossible odds, simply because many families want assurance that they have "tried everything," without weighing the burdens and suffering involved. In one study, 32% of the surrogates who were given a prognosis of less than a 1% survival rate asked for life support to be continued (Zier et al., 2009).

Nurses view this through an ethics of caring lens both because of their training and their close proximity to patients, placing them at high risk for recurrent moral distress. When nurses still have their souls intact, there is moral outrage at resuscitating a child who is within hours of dying, all because the parents are in denial or unable to shoulder the burden of saying enough is enough. Or the nurse might be caring for a cancer patient in multiorgan failure with metastatic disease who has sustained a stroke, has sepsis, and is now ventilated, with a family requesting dialysis for the renal failure.

The preciousness of life valued by our society accounts for the extraordinary effort made to prolong it. However, aggressive treatments not only extend dying, but ultimately beget an appalling disintegration of the body and person. A nurse with her conscience intact is left asking hard questions, as she is constrained from doing what she believes is right: to do no harm. Additionally, when the nurse steps away from the individual bedside, she is also acutely aware of the justice issues in health care. Whether the pitiable lack of mental health resources or the limited supports for patients dying in their homes, there is an ache for what is spent for the one and not for the other.

What can be done as we attempt to balance the needs of individual values and technology, that advances medicine, yet is also reminiscent of Pandora's Box? How can appropriate professional goals of treatment be addressed in our multicultural and multifaith society? Policies must be developed and used that address non-beneficial treatment. "Death panels" must give way to open forums where the public begins to see the aberrant behavior of health care teams providing harmful treatments that are powerless in the face of death. The courts must join the difficult debates and shoulder some of the responsibility for balancing patient rights with limitations of treatment. The most vulnerable in our society must be assured a just process.

Ultimately, there is an ethical obligation for our society to conserve the health care dollars that are driving our country into debt; the national debate must think in terms of justice that allows for financial parity. Even in the care of the dying, there is inequity that permits millions to be spent on a dying patient in an intensive care unit, while limiting hospice care in the home to under $200 per day. Righting this disparity would not only improve end-stage care for many, it would also decrease immense amounts of suffering.

Nurses are often aware of early indications of ethical conflicts and, given adequate ethics education, they can be in a prime position for setting a process in motion before issues escalate (Pavlish, Brown-Saltzman, Hersh, Shirk, & Nudelman, 2011). They are also excellent candidates for obtaining degrees in bioethics: with their clinical knowledge, they can elucidate these issues in powerful ways.

discussion point

Do you have moral courage? Would you report an impaired physician? Would you administer a medication you knew to be an error because you knew the physician would go off on you for refusing?

It's your turn ... start the discussion!

_____

_____

_____

_____

_____

_____

_____

_____

_____

Our institutions must make a commitment to create moral environments that encourage and listen to these voices, from the questions that are asked during the hiring process to making sure that ethics consultation is available and promoted as a routine part of care. We know from research that one action that changes the escalation of moral distress is for nurses to speak out when their inner voices tell them that "something is not right" (Epstein & Hamric, 2009).

—**Katherine Brown-Saltzman**, _MA, RN, is co-director of the UCLA Health System Ethics Center._

References

American Association of Critical Care Nurses. (2006). *Moral distress.* Retrieved from http://www.aacn.org/WD/Practice/Docs/Moral_Distress.pdf

Caldwell, E. S., Lu, H., & Harding, T. (2010). Encompassing multiple moral paradigms: A challenge for nursing educators. *Nursing Ethics, 17,* 189-199.

Corley, M. C. (2002). Nurse moral distress: A proposed theory and research agenda. *Nursing Ethics, 9,* 636-650.

Dierckx de Casterlé, B., Izumi, S., Godfrey, N. S., & Denhaerynck, K. (2008). Nurses' responses to ethical dilemmas in nursing practice: Meta-analysis. *Journal of Advanced Nursing, 63,* 540-549.

Epstein, E. G., & Hamric, A. B. (2009). Moral distress, moral residue, and the crescendo effect. *The Journal of Clinical Ethics, 20*(4), 330-334.

Institute of Medicine. (2011). *The future of nursing: Leading change, advancing health.* Retrieved from http://www.iom.edu/Reports/2010/The-Future-of-Nursing-Leading-Change-Advancing-Health.aspx

Kain, V. (2007). Moral distress and providing care to dying babies in neonatal nursing. *International Journal of Palliative Nursing, 13,* 243-248.

McCarthy, J., & Deady, R. (2008). Moral distress reconsidered. *Nursing Ethics, 15,* 254-262.

Olmstead, D. L., Scott, S. D., & Austin, W. J. (2010). Unresolved pain in children: A relational ethics perspective. *Nursing Ethics, 17,* 695-704.

Pavlish, C., Brown-Saltzman, K., Hersh, M., Shirk, M., & Nudelman, O. (2011). Early indicators and risk factors for ethical issues in clinical practice. *Journal of Nursing Scholarship.* doi:10.1111/j.1547-5069.2010.01380.x

Ramsey, D. J., Schmidt, M. L., & Sanderson-Shaw, L. (2010). Online ethics discussion forum facilitates medical center clinical ethics case reviews. *JONA's Healthcare Law, Ethics, and Regulation, 12,* 15-20.

Robinson, R. (2010). Registered nurses and moral distress. *Dimensions in Critical Care Nursing, 29,* 197-202.

Ulrich, C. M., & Hamric, A. B. (2008). What is so distressing about moral distress in advanced practice nursing? *Clinical Scholars Review, 1*, 5-6.

Ulrich, C. M., O'Donnell, P., Taylor, C., Farrar, A., Danis, M., & Grady, C. (2007). Ethical climate, ethics stress, and the job satisfaction of nurses and social workers in the United States. *Social Science and Medicine, 65*(8), 1708-1719.

U.S. Census Bureau. (2010). *Aging boomers will increase dependency ratio*. U.S. Census Bureau Projects.

Wocial, L. D., Hancock, M., Bledsoe, P. D., & Chamness, A. R. (2010). An evaluation of unit-based ethics conversations. *JONA's Healthcare Law, Ethics, and Regulation, 12*, 48-54.

Wright, D., & Brajtman, S. (2011). Relational and embodied knowing: Nursing ethics with the interprofessional team. *Nursing Ethics, 18*, 20-30.

Zier, L. S., Burack, J. H., Micco, G., Chipman, A.K., Frank, J. A., Luce, J. M., & White, D. B. (2009). Surrogate decision makers' responses to physicians' predictions of medical futility. Chest, 136(1), 110-117.

Question #7:

How Do We Fix the Workplace Culture of Nursing?

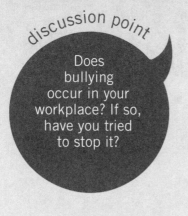

For decades, we've heard the old saw "nurses eat their young," and most have experienced it firsthand. Sure, there's sometimes doctor-on-nurse bullying or patient-on-nurse violence, but the real issue is nurses—women—who bully each other. Finally, after years of high turnover and young nurses leaving the profession, nurse leaders and researchers are starting to pay attention.

So what is going on? Let's face it: There are still some older nurses who feel like the younger ones should "pay their dues." Bullying can be rooted in cultural or racial issues. It's present in academia and among faculty, and even found in old-fashioned cliques among women. It's not that different from what any of us may have experienced in the school yard.

But health care environments are more complicated than the school yard. There are seriously ill or injured patients, crushing workloads, and distressed families. No, being a nurse is not easy, but neither is it an excuse for bad behavior.

It is time for every nurse to honestly examine and evaluate his or her own behavior toward coworkers and acknowledge if he or she is, in fact, a bully. As nurses, don't we want to stop this? Instead of denying it exists, let's start a conversation about how we can turn it around.

Working Together to Change Nursing's Culture

by Fay Bower

There are 3 million nurses in the United States (Institute of Medicine, 2011). But these nurses are not all "on the same page" when it comes to agreeing on some key nursing issues, such as the current debate about the DNP role or the entry to practice with a BSN degree. To improve the way in which nurses treat one another within the profession, the first step is to convince all nurses there is a need to come together as one large and potentially strong voice.

If we want more consensus within the profession, nursing leaders and state and national professional organizations must work together more consistently. It was a proud moment to see all of the major professional nursing organizations come together to support the Institute of Medicine (IOM) recommendations. This needs to occur more often.

To improve the profession's culture, there must also be a change in the relationship between education and practice. When I became a nurse, I was greeted with open arms, as I was prepared in a hospital program and thus was one of the hospital's workforce from day one. I was welcomed and mentored. I worked on the unit every day and went to school in the hospital every evening.

What do you think?

_____

_____

_____

_____

_____

_____

_____

_____

_____

_____

_____

Did you know …

In a report from the Joint Commission …

"Effective January 1, 2009, the Joint Commission promulgated a new Leadership Standard (LD. 03.01.01 to address intimidating, disruptive, and inappropriate behaviors. The Joint Commission cited research demonstrating that negative interpersonal conduct by physicians and others can lead to medical errors, preventable adverse patient outcomes, poor patient satisfaction, increased cost of care, increased malpractice risk, and turnover among professionals who have to deal with the abusive offenders" (Crisis Prevention Institute, 2008, para. 2).

Today, most nursing students are educated in the college or university setting and spend much less time in the hospital. This division of education from practice has made it difficult for educators and staff to unite around professional issues. This needs to change. Having faculty and staff working together on curriculum, students spending time in residency programs, and staff being included in the classroom could move the personal culture of nursing in a different direction.

Can the four generations of nurses work together? They must if the profession is to survive. While the values and expectations are somewhat different for each generation, the goals and objectives of nursing (caring, promoting health, and preventing illness) provide the framework for the practice of nursing, which includes differences. Acceptance of differences is the key to making it possible to work together. So again, the challenge is to learn how to accept another's beliefs and to make an effort to include them in the care of patients and in everyday activities with colleagues.

The barriers to these changes rest within each nurse. Nurse leaders and nursing organizations must step up remove these barriers.

—**Fay Bower**, *DNSc, FAAN, is professor and chair of nursing at Holy Names University in Oakland, California, USA, and a past president of the Honor Society of Nursing, Sigma Theta Tau International.*

Diversity Transforms Nursing's Professional Culture

by Ken Dion

Changing demographics and economics will have a large impact on the professional culture of nursing during the next 3 years. The demographics referred to are not those of the aging U.S. population, but changes within the profession itself. A once Caucasian, female-dominated profession is rapidly becoming more ethnically and gender diverse with nurses who are working at nearly all points of the life span, from the "Millennials" to the "veteran generation."

Nurses of diverse ethnic origins will bring an interpretation of caring, the essence of nursing, to the profession that has been shaped by their upbringing and ethnicity. These influences—such as therapeutic touch, meditation, guide visualization, and other holistic interventions—in many cases are more closely aligned with the founding principles of the nursing profession than we sometimes see in Western medicine.

More men are entering the profession because of its employment security. They, too, bring their own interpretation of caring. Moreover, men are socialized differently from women during their formative years and therefore will undoubtedly influence the profession's personal culture. However, in my experience, men are no less caring than their female counterparts and, as such, their sometimes

Top 10 challenges

"[We need to avoid] glorifying credentials over contributions."

–**Sarah H. Kagan**, PhD, RN, Lucy Walker Honorary Term Professor of Gerontological Nursing and clinical nurse specialist, Abramson Cancer Center, University of Pennsylvania, USA

Top 10 challenges

"Start taking responsibility for the way we relate to ourselves."

–**Kathleen Heinrich**, PhD, RN, principal, KTH Consulting, Guilford, Connecticut, USA

Did you know ...

While everyone may be able to provide his or her own definition of respect, a survey of RNs conducted by the Respect Project (Ulrich, Breugger, & Lefton, 2009) identified the following five behaviors that indicate respect and will help you rise above a difficult situation:

1. Listen, be fully attentive, and truly hear.

2. Acknowledge and express appreciation.

3. Exhibit empathy and understanding.

4. Display courtesy and consideration.

5. Be accountable and professional.

different style of delivering care will serve to enhance the profession both internally and with the public.

The profession will see a decline in its numbers when the baby boomers begin to retire. The younger nurses who will be filling their shoes were raised in a prosperous macroeconomic time. This fact manifests itself in different expectations of the relationship with their employer, the work environment, and the opportunities within the profession. If properly funded and implemented, interventions such as nurse residencies—recommended by the National Council of State Boards of Nursing, the Robert Wood Johnson Foundation, and others—will assist in decreasing the transition shock often experienced by younger graduates that results in high turnover and exits from the profession. Furthermore, implementation of residencies will support the transfer of knowledge from one generation to the next by those with a desire to educate their colleagues, rather than those forced to precept. Through this transitional process, the younger nurses who remain will hopefully share a common affinity for caring, the calling that drew their predecessors to the profession.

How do we change the profession's personal culture? By focusing on the promotion of diversity of all kinds within the nursing ranks. Achieving this goal will be difficult without mobilizing our society to demand a health care system that emphasizes the importance of nursing in delivering optimal patient care, because resources to do so will remain scarce. Four generations should easily agree that caring for our fellow man is the reason why we enter the profession of nursing.

—**Ken Dion**, *PhD, MSN, MBA, RN, is founder and CEO of Decision Critical.*

Generational Diversity in the Workplace: Vive la différence!

by Carol J. Huston

Much has been written about generational diversity in nursing over the past decade, perhaps because in the past, three and even four generations typically did not work together in a profession at the same time (Huston, in press). Current research suggests that such diversity may present challenges, because different generations of nurses often have dissimilar values and ways of thinking. This diversity provides opportunities, however, for intergenerational partnerships and multiple perspectives that result in the best thinking.

A review of the literature, which is rapidly becoming a global body of knowledge, suggests that four generational groups are usually identified in the current nursing workforce: the veteran generation (also called the silent generation), baby boomers, Generation X, and Generation Y (also called the Millennials).

The veteran generation is typically recognized as those born between 1925 and 1942 (Huston, in press). Having lived through several international military conflicts—World War II, the Korean War and Vietnam—and the Great Depression, they may be more risk-averse (particularly in regard to personal finances), respectful of authority, supportive of hierarchy and disciplined (Patterson, 2007).

Veterans are also called the silent generation, because they tend to support the status quo rather than protest or push for rapid change. As a result, nurses from

discussion point

OK, be honest: Is there a time when you've been the bully? Have you gotten frustrated with someone who is new? Have you explained the procedure already and they're still not getting it? Meanwhile, you're falling behind in your work. We've all been there. Think of a situation, and then name three techniques that you could try to change it.

this generation are less likely to question organizational practices and more likely to seek employment in structured settings (Marquis & Huston, 2009). Their work values also tend to be more traditional, and they are often recognized for loyalty to their employers.

The boom generation (born 1943-1964) also displays traditional work values. However, baby boomers tend to be more materialistic and thus willing to work long hours in an effort to get ahead (Huston, in press). Indeed, workers of this generation are more apt than any other to be called workaholics, and their general inclination is to live for the present rather than the future (Patterson, 2007). This generation is also recognized as being more individualistic, which often results in greater creativity and a tendency to challenge rules. Thus, nurses of this generation may be best suited for work that requires flexibility, independent thinking and creativity.

In contrast, Generation Xers (born between 1963 and 1983) may lack interest in lifetime employment at one place, a custom that prior generations valued. Instead, they value flexible work hours and opportunities for time off. Thus, this generation may be less driven economically than prior generations and may define success differently than the veteran generation or baby boomers. Research by Leiter, Jackson and Shaughnessy (2009) suggests that these value differences may contribute to a greater mismatch between personal and organizational values for Generation X nurses than for baby boomer nurses. This mismatch is associated with greater susceptibility to burn out and a stronger inclination for Generation X nurses to quit. At the same time, Generation Xers are pragmatic, self-reliant and amenable to change (Patterson, 2007).

Generation Y (born between1980 and 2001) includes the profession's youngest nurses and represents the first cohort of truly global citizens (Huston, in press). They are known for optimism, self-confidence, relationship-orientation, volunteer-mindedness and social consciousness. They are also highly sophisticated in the use of technology, which allows them to view the world as a "smaller, diverse, highly networked environment in which to work and live" (Patterson, 2007, p. 20). Thus, people comprising this generation are often called "digital natives." Generation Y workers do, however, frequently demand a different type of organizational culture to meet their needs (Piper, 2008). In fact, Generation Y nurses may test the patience of their baby boomer leaders, since they may "come with a sense of entitlement that can be an affront to older workers. They want to do something meaningful today" (What does it take, para. 6).

Mensik (2004) suggests that, although generational diversity poses new management challenges, it also provides a variety of perspectives and outlooks that enhance workplace balance and productivity. She notes that the literature often focuses on negative attributes and differences between the generations, particularly for Generation X and Generation Y, and that a more balanced view is needed. For example, the literature repeatedly indicates that these age groups may have less loyalty to their employers than the generations that preceded them, but Mensik cites current research suggesting that commitment to employment longevity is actually greater for Generation X and Generation Y than for the boomers who preceded them (Huston, in press).

Top 10 challenges

"Prepare all nurses to channel their passion for practice into presentations, publications, and research that get the word out about the challenges facing us, not least of which is ourselves."

–Kathleen Heinrich, PhD, RN, principal, KTH Consulting, Guilford, Connecticut, USA

Top 10 challenges

"[It is a challenge that nursing professionals are unable] to act and work together cohesively. [We have become a] fractionated profession that has limited professional power."

–Carol L. Huston, DPA, MSN, MPA, FAAN, director, School of Nursing, California State University, Chico, California, USA

Top 10 challenges

"Take responsibility for the way we treat others, whether we are in practice, education, or leadership."

–Kathleen Heinrich, PhD, RN, principal, KTH Consulting, Guilford, Connecticut, USA

Top 10 challenges

"[We need to] stop blaming others for incivility threatening to destroy the caring essence of our profession."

"Start taking responsibility for the way we relate to ourselves."

–Kathleen Heinrich, PhD, RN, principal, KTH Consulting, Guilford, Connecticut, USA

Top 10 challenges

"[Nurses need to] refuse to participate in joy-stealing games that splinter self-esteem and fracture relationships, e.g. The Shame Game, The Devalue Game, The Splitting Game, etc."

–Kathleen Heinrich, PhD, RN, principal, KTH Consulting, Guilford, Connecticut, USA

Mensik (2004) concludes that, instead of focusing on generational differences, nurses should move forward and put their energies into seeking collaboration among generations. Patients benefit from the optimal outcomes that occur when all generations work together as a high-performing team (Huston, in press).

Boivin (2008) agrees and observes that patients benefit the most from differences and strengths among nurses. This diversity, she argues, allows patients to "have nurses caring for them who have 20 or 30 years' experience under their belts, who are able to use the latest technology to prevent errors, and who are willing to challenge authority and act as patient advocates" (para. 14). Finally, Thomas (2007) suggests that fostering generational partnerships is absolutely critical in nursing to ensure transference of knowledge from retiring baby boomers to newer generations of nurses.

Clearly, generational diversity in nursing should be viewed positively, as each generation brings unique characteristics, experiences, skill sets and perspectives to the profession. By focusing on commonalities as well as appreciating and valuing our differences, intergenerational partnerships in nursing should provide new opportunities to collaborate to improve global health.

Reprinted from Reflections on Nursing Leadership, *Vol. 35, No. 2.*

—**Carol J. Huston**, *DPA, MSN, MPA, FAAN, is director of the School of Nursing at California State University in Chico, California, USA, and a past president of the Honor Society of Nursing, Sigma Theta Tau International.*

References

Boivin, J. (2008, August 11). Opinion. Nursing enters a new era. Four generations healing under one hospital roof. *Nursing Spectrum. NurseWeek.* Retrieved 11 August 2008 from http://include.nurse.com/apps/pbcs.dll/article?AID=/20080811/FL02/308110018

Crisis Prevention Institute. (2008). *The Joint Commission Leadership Standard (LD.03.01.01) addressing disruptive and inappropriate behaviors/The CPI Workplace Bullying seminar.* Retrieved from http://www.crisisprevention.com/CPI/media/Media/Resources/alignments/Joint-Commission-Workplace-Bullying-Alignment-2011.pdf

Huston, C. (in press). Diversity in the nursing workforce. In C. Huston (Ed.), *Professional issues in nursing* (2nd ed.). Philadelphia: Lippincott Williams & Wilkins.

Institute of Medicine. (2011). *The future of nursing. Leading change, advancing health.* Washington, DC: The National Academies Press.

It's your turn ... start the discussion!

_____

_____

_____

_____

_____

_____

_____

_____

_____

_____

_____

_____

Leiter, M.P., Jackson, N.J., & Shaughnessy, K. (2009, January). Contrasting burnout, turnover intention, control, value congruence and knowledge sharing between Baby Boomers and Generation X. *Journal of Nursing Management, 17*(1), 100-109.

Marquis, B., & Huston, C. (2009). *Leadership roles and management functions in nursing* (6th ed.). Philadelphia: Lippincott Williams & Wilkins.

Mensik, J. S. (November 2007). A view on generational differences from a generation X leader. *Journal of Nursing Administration, 37*(11), 483-484.

Patterson, C.K. (2007). The impact of generational diversity in the workplace. *Diversity Factor, 15*(3), 17-22.

Piper, L.E. (April-June 2008). The Generation-Y workforce in health care: The new challenge for leadership. *Health Care Manager, 27*(2), 98-103.

Thomas, J.M. (2007). Creating roles to retain the experienced mature nurse in the post-anesthesia care unit. *Perioperative Nursing Clinics, 2*(4), 337-344. Retrieved 14 March 2009 from http://www.periopnursing.theclinics.com/article/S1556-7931(07)00076-9/abstract

Ulrich, B., Breugger, R., & Lefton, C. (2009). *Respect: Beginning to define the concept in nursing.* Retrieved from http://www.navigatenursing.org/PDFs/article%20nurses%20first%20defining%20respect.pdf

What does it take to build bridges among the different generations? (2008, April). *OR Manager, 24*(4), 10.

Question #8:

What Role Do Nurse Leaders Play in the Profession?

Top 10 challenges

"[The profession needs] further collaborative efforts between other health care providers and nursing to continue to function as a team effort for the welfare of the patient. Sometimes I feel we are losing ground in this critical area."

–**Vicki Michelle McMahon**, MSN, RN

Of the key messages and recommendations of the Institute of Medicine's much-discussed report on the future of nursing, the one that may be the most difficult to implement is the call for the transformation of nursing leadership.

Two short lines in the report indicate why. Those lines say that most nurses entering the profession do not envision themselves as future leaders, and that the public—although holding nurses in high regard—is not used to seeing them as leaders (Institute of Medicine, 2011).

It's a chicken-egg effect. If nurses do not view themselves as leaders, then how can they convince the public and their health care colleagues that they are indeed leaders who should be respected and listened to?

The report goes on to say that nurse leaders need to be cultivated and nurtured from the bedside to the boardroom in order for nurses to achieve key message #3: Nurses need to be full partners with physicians and other health professionals in redesigning health care in the United States.

If you are already a nurse leader and do not encourage your nurses to think and act like leaders, it's time to start the discussion.

Nourishing Future Leaders

by Carol Picard

One of the most important things current nursing leaders can do is to cultivate, nourish, and sustain future leaders. It is a moral obligation we have to the future of our profession. Future leaders must be nourished from the moment they enter nursing as students. Faculty can "call out" the innate capacities they see in students by telling them what they observe. Whenever I work with students who have leadership traits, I encourage them to take advantage of early opportunities to get involved at school, in the first nursing positions and, of course, in voluntary organizations.

Sharing wisdom learned with young leaders can give them a vision for their own future. Here are some thoughts I share as I speak with them. Personal development is at the heart of my message.

First, have a vision. How will you leave your fingerprints on this profession? This is your point of engagement with others to articulate what you believe is possible.

Listen to and show respect for different points of view. Strength can come from learning to debate an issue and in understanding those who do not agree with us.

discussion point

What is the difference between a leader and a manager?

Did you know ...

For the first time, the NLC (2011 Nursing Leadership Congress) included a day of clinical leadership collaboration with physician peers. Attendees participated in an interactive table discussion on how to achieve high reliability through strategic communication, collaboration models, and the use of technology.

"A transformed system will need nurses with the adaptive capacity to take on reconceptualized roles in new settings, educating and reeducating themselves along the way—indispensible characteristics of effective leadership" (Institute of Medicine, 2011, p. 32).

Third, learn from your mistakes. The goal is to not make the same mistake twice, but to glean from root cause analysis what led to your mistake. It can also be helpful to share this experience with others in selected situations. I will never forget being at a Schwartz Center Rounds at Massachusetts General Hospital where the chief of oncology began the meeting sharing a mistake he had made. It gave permission to others present in the room to consider their own mistakes and how to talk about them with colleagues.

Also, be willing to share the credit for your success. The strongest leaders make sure credit is shared with others. Keep your finger on the pulse of the organization. Joyce Clifford, eminent nurse leader of one of the first hospitals identified as a Magnet for nurses, is an example of a leader who paid close attention to and gave support to what was happening to nurses at the bedside.

Time spent in reflection for self-awareness and dialogue with mentors will help you to recognize your weaknesses as well as strengths. Leadership has its frustrations. Actively work to let go of negative emotions. If you keep a balance by nourishing your inner life and your personal relationships, you will have more energy available to dedicate to who you are as a nursing leader.

The love of the profession, the courage to live up to your potential, and the ability to honor those who surround you are pillars for leaders past, present, and future.

—**Carol Picard**, *PhD, RN, is president of Carol Picard Associates and past president of the Honor Society of Nursing, Sigma Theta Tau International.*

Strengthening Nursing Through Responsibility and Advocacy

by Rebecca M. Patton

"For us who Nurse, our Nursing is a thing, which, unless in it we are making progress every year, every month, every week, take my word for it, we are going back."

—*Florence Nightingale*

How true those words are today. With the recent pro-nursing, pro-patient legislative successes—particularly in the Affordable Care Act—our profession is positioned favorably. The latest Institute of Medicine (2011) report, *The Future of Nursing: Leading Change, Advancing Health*, has been viewed as optimistic for our profession. So it is not surprising to hear many say, "This is nursing's time. The stars are aligned for us."

Well, what does that actually mean and, more importantly, will it last? Nurses are being recognized as independent providers of health care and working as equal partners with other practitioners. Advanced practice registered nurses (APRNs) are benefiting with improved recognition, compensation, and reimbursement. Individuals are pursing APRN roles versus going into medicine. However, we know that this is not sufficient, nor what is required so that every patient encounter is safe, free of harm, compassionate, and of the highest quality possible.

Top 10 challenges

"[What is] the leadership role of the nurse in the health care team? Can the nurse lead when the doctors are around? This is a big issue in our setting."

—**Mary Opare**, MSN, DipEd, RN, acting dean of nursing and senior lecturer, University of Ghana, Legon, Republic of Ghana, West Africa

Did you know …

"The new style of leadership that is needed flows in all directions at all levels. Everyone from the bedside to the boardroom must engage colleagues, subordinates, and executives so that together they can identify and achieve common goals" (Bradford & Cohen, 1998, as cited in Institute of Medicine, 2011, p. 223).

Our profession has several unforgiving realities. We are not always in control of our practice. We are not the decision makers or influential where we ought to be. We do not receive the respect we earn. And, most importantly, we have not leveraged the strength we are capable of engineering. As nurses, we are intelligent, highly skillful, ethical individuals with a driven passion, and we endure physically and mentally when others would give up.

So what is needed to strengthen our profession? Not just to achieve a particular goal, but so that we persevere and give rise to meaningful impact and influence in our society on all matters of importance? We need to start at the beginning, with the education and the socialization to become a registered nurse. Lesson number one is responsibility and advocacy for the profession. Inspire the value of a strong profession, and do not get distracted by diversity of opinions that has only splintered our strengths and created barriers.

As airlines demonstrate on every flight, put the oxygen mask on yourself first, so that you can take care of others. Our ability to achieve for others often has been lessened with the lack of personal responsibility and advocacy for our profession. While we can learn the skills to collaborate and communicate, and everything else, the value of personal responsibility is integral to our enduring ability to lead and achieve.

—**Rebecca M. Patton**, *MSN, RN, CNOR, FAAN, is Atkinson Visiting Instructor in Perioperative Nursing at Frances Payne Bolton School of Nursing, Case Western Reserve University, and immediate past president of the American Nurses Association.*

Advancing Nursing Through the Practice Environment

by Jeanette Ives Erickson

In today's complex health care environment, nurse leaders are faced with the challenge of strengthening the nursing profession within their organizations and across the care-delivery system. Improving the professional practice environment is the best place for chief nursing officers (CNO) to focus their efforts in advancing the discipline and science of nursing. CNOs need to explain the concept and status of the practice environment to superiors, peers, and subordinates to help advance the profession.

Florence Nightingale (1859), the founder of modern nursing, was the first to talk about the importance of the total healing environment. Nightingale's work had a momentous influence on the fundamental values of healthy work environments (Ives Erickson, 2010) and has been echoed by every major professional nursing organization. Still, many CNOs today do not effectively articulate the practice environment as the rallying point for advancing nursing (Adams, Ives Erickson, Jones, & Paulo, 2009).

While no singular definition of the practice environment exists, practice-environment measurement instruments have been developed. One description of the professional practice environment includes the core components of autonomy, clinician-MD relations, control over practice, cultural sensitivity, teamwork,

Top 10 challenges

"Support the principles of a 'Magnet' culture and environment for nurses in all practice settings where the expectation is excellence and the organization has prioritized the nursing profession and supports this approach. It necessitates the presence and organizational authority of a strong nurse leader in developing a business case for resources and a presence at the table for decision-making."

—**Karen Hill**, DNP, RN, NEA-BC, vice president and nurse executive, Central Baptist Hospital, Lexington, Kentucky, USA

It's your turn ... start the discussion!

----

communication, conflict-management, and internal work motivation (Ives Erickson et al., 2004; Adams et al., 2009). Based on this framework, evidence indicates that the practice environment of nurses is significantly related to organizational, patient, and professional outcomes: Positive practice environments lead to positive outcomes.

Measuring and understanding staff nurse perceptions of the professional practice environment must be core responsibilities of the CNO and all nurse leaders. A CNO views the world through the lens of improving the environment in which care is delivered. The CNO develops empowered nurses who advance nursing and develop the next generation of leaders.

Articulating a professional practice model and evaluating that model are linked processes. Neither is ever complete; they always inform the other. Both processes fuel the CNO's power in the organization. Power, as proposed by Elizabeth Barrett (1989), is the capacity to participate knowingly in the nature of change, characterizing the continuous mutual process of people and their world. The measurable dimensions of power are awareness, choices, freedom to act intentionally, and involvement in creating change (Barrett, 1989). As new care-delivery models unfold, having a mechanism to inform the CNO about what's working and, more importantly, what's not working, positions the CNO to participate knowingly in shaping the future of care-delivery.

—**Jeanette Ives Erickson**, *MS, RN, FAAN, is senior vice president for patient care and chief nurse at Massachusetts General Hospital, Boston; assistant professor at Massachusetts General Hospital Institute of Health Professions; instructor at Harvard Medical School; visiting scholar at Boston College; and senior associate at The Institute for Nursing Healthcare Leadership.*

References

Adams, J.M., Ives Erickson, J., Jones, D.A., & Paulo, L. (2009). An evidence based structure for transformative nurse executive practice: The Model of the Interrelationship of Leadership, Environments & Outcomes for Nurse Executives (MILE ONE), *Nursing Administration Quarterly, 33*(4), 280-287.

Barrett, E.A.M. (1989). A nursing theory of power for nursing practice: Derivation from Rogers' paradigm. In J. Riehl (Ed.), Conceptual models for nursing practice (3rd ed.) (pp. 207-217). Norwalk, CT: Appleton & Lange.

Bradford, D.L., & Cohen, A.R. (1998). *Power up: Transforming organizations through shared leadership.* Hoboken, NJ: John Wiley & Sons.

Institute of Medicine. (2011). *The future of nursing: Leading change, advancing health.* Washington, DC: National Academies Press.

Ives Erickson, J. (2010, January 31). Overview and summary: Promoting healthy work environments: A shared responsibility. *OJIN: The Online Journal of Issues in Nursing, 15*(1), Manuscript Overview.

Ives Erickson, J., Duffy, M., Gibbons, M., Fitzmaurice, J., Ditomassi, M., & Jones, D. (2004). Development and psychometric evaluation of the professional practice environment (PPE) scale. *Journal of Nursing Scholarship, 6*(3), 279-285.

Nightingale, F. (1859). *Notes on nursing: What it is and what it is not.* (1st American edition). New York: Appleton and Company.

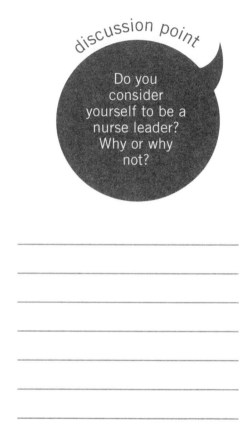

discussion point

Do you consider yourself to be a nurse leader? Why or why not?

Notes

_____
_____
_____
_____
_____
_____
_____
_____
_____
_____
_____

Question #9:

What Are We Going to Do About the Widening Workforce Age Gap?

Top 10 challenges

"[One of the biggest challenges is] having to prepare very rapidly for an aging society."

–**Sarah H. Kagan**, PhD, RN, Lucy Walker Honorary Term Professor of Gerontological Nursing and clinical nurse specialist, Abramson Cancer Center, University of Pennsylvania, USA

When it comes to age, the real question is how an aging—and soon-to-be retiring—workforce is going to handle the increasing number of elderly. Seriously, what is our plan to handle all these older people? In the not-so-distant future, we are going to be the ones called "old" by our younger counterparts! Nurses already notching into their 50s can only hope that robots are not wiping their or their patients' mouths or putting them into a bathtub of hot water 20 years down the road. (Yes, there really is an experiment now taking place in Japan, and according to a news report on the study from the BBC, the island's over-65 set isn't exactly thrilled about the metallic caregivers.)

So, what happens when an aging workforce is well on its way to becoming the aging population? The 2008 National Sample Survey of Registered Nurses (USDHHS, 2010) reports the average age of a nurse is 46. Other reports show a median age of nurses as high as 55. Maybe it's time to start asking who is going to take care of us—never mind the rest of the population—if younger nurses don't start making up a larger percentage of the profession and taking more of an interest in learning about the care of older adults.

Unfortunately, most nurses don't gravitate to gerontology. Gero patients often have chronic problems and are facing other issues, such as losing their independence and mental capacity. It's just not as sexy or fulfilling as acute care, trauma, or pediatrics.

Additionally, faculty shortages have made it difficult to get into nursing school, and the current number of graduates isn't enough to fill the widening gap. Maybe it's time to start the conversation and develop a new framework about how we're going to care for the aging in America. If we can't, when it's your turn, that robot may be looking pretty good.

If We Could See Through Their Eyes

by Claudia K.Y. Lai

In 1994, I started to study dementia and the care of people with that disorder. I did so simply because a professor of a master's course I was taking specializes in dementia care. I have been interested in the care of older people for a long time. I worked in a rehabilitation and chronic care hospital while I was studying for my baccalaureate degree. Due to the nature of the services that particular hospital provided, a large proportion of the patients were older adults. That was where my interest in elder care began to grow.

As one requirement for this master's course, the professor asked us to spend a day in a nursing home, trying out the nursing assessment tool she had shown us. After arriving at the home, we dispersed and I went into a resident's room. The occupant, an elderly lady, agreed to speak with me. I must confess that I do not recall

> ### Top 10 challenges
>
> *"[We need to face] issues related to gerontology and long-term care challenges."*
>
> **–Daniel J. Pesut,** PhD, RN, PMHCNS-BC, FAAN, professor, Indiana University School of Nursing, Indianapolis, Indiana, USA

discussion point

Do you have experience in gero nursing? Why did you take the job? Name three things you liked and three things you disliked about it.

_____

_____

_____

_____

_____

_____

asking for her consent before assessing her. Anyway, we started, and I asked her to follow my instructions—to raise an arm, to raise both arms, and so on and so forth.

After three or four commands, she looked at me and asked, "Are you testing me?" That was one of the more awkward moments in my professional life. I didn't know much about dementia back then. How I related to people with dementia was governed by assumptions and ignorance. I thought that people who suffered from dementia would not know what I was doing. Her response caught me by surprise. I felt terrible for testing this lady, who had the insight to appreciate what was happening.

However, it was also one of the most memorable moments in my professional life. I became acutely aware that, in fact, all these tests we professionals are so proud of mastering mean very little to the people who, either voluntarily or involuntarily, become the subjects of our testing.

Following this incident, all of the assignments for my master's program focused on different issues related to dementia care, and I realized that there was a great deal of literature on the care of *caregivers* of people with dementia, but very little on those unfortunate enough to suffer from the disease.

As I traveled along the road of my academic career, I immersed myself in writing grant proposals, developing networks, conducting research projects and preparing manuscripts. The field of dementia care is very much multidisciplinary. I became disillusioned after seeing that the work of the various disciplines—nursing included—did not always meet the needs of people with dementia and their loved ones.

As researchers and clinicians, we are all very keen to develop new measures and interventions, and to study their effects over time. But do people with dementia need all these assessments and interventions? I tried to visualize myself as a dementia patient, with all of these experiments performed on me. And I knew that, if I were suffering from dementia, I would want researchers and clinicians, first and foremost, to appreciate the kind of person I am and plan my care accordingly. I knew I would want some peace.

Adapted from Reflections on Nursing Leadership, *Vol. 36, No. 2.*

–**Claudia Kam Yuk Lai,** *PhD, RN, is a professor in the School of Nursing at Hong Kong Polytechnic University, Hong Kong SAR, China. Her specialty is gerontological nursing.*

What do you think?

Top 10
challenges

"[Think about] the loss of nursing wisdom and leadership due to retirements and poor (or nonexistent) succession planning and mentoring of next generation leaders."

—**Daniel J. Pesut**, PhD, RN, PMHCNS-BC, FAAN, professor, Indiana University School of Nursing, Indianapolis, Indiana, USA

The Tsunami of an Aging Nation

by Tara Cortes

With 77 million baby boomers beginning to turn 65 years old in 2011, coupled with the advances being made in science, the number of people over age 65 is expected to increase from 30 million to more than 70 million by 2025. These statistics set the stage for a health care crisis. We do not have an adequate workforce prepared to meet the specialized needs of older adults in the years to come.

Two significant events in 2010 will shape the way we meet this impending crisis. On March 23, 2010, President Obama signed into law the Patient Protection and Affordable Care Act, which expands health care coverage to an additional 32 million people. Although this health care reform act is not specific to older adults, it does include specific programs to increase the capacity of the health care workforce to care for the aging population.

In October 2010, The Institute of Medicine released a groundbreaking, comprehensive analysis of the nursing profession, *The Future of Nursing: Leading Change, Advancing Health*. The report recognizes the role of nursing in patient-centered care, including primary care and care coordination across all settings for older adults.

These documents open the way for RNs and advanced practice registered nurses (APRNs) to play a major role in the care of older adults. The knowledge explosion has rendered us a society of super specialty health care providers, and in this paradigm APRNs are essential for the future of primary care. There is evidence that APRNs are effective in managing chronic disease and maintaining function in patients. Nurses have demonstrated their ability to coordinate care amongst a team of providers. These nurses can provide comprehensive primary care and refer to specialists and other professionals as appropriate.

In order to be effective in this role, nurses need expert knowledge in caring for the specialized needs of older adults. Educational programs need to ensure their graduates have adequate preparation. Practice settings must appropriately reinforce this knowledge. The John A. Hartford Foundation has been instrumental in supporting an infrastructure to promote these activities. We need to know that APRNs use evidence-based practice to manage chronic diseases and maintain optimal function. Models that create opportunities for nurses to coordinate safe transitions for older adults across the health care continuum are essential. Nurses can be instrumental in shaping quality care for older adults.

—**Tara A. Cortes**, *PhD, RN, FAAN, is executive director of The Hartford Institute for Geriatric Nursing and professor of geriatric nursing at New York University College of Nursing in New York.*

> ## Top 10 challenges
>
> *"[It's time to address] the aging nursing workforce, both in academia and service areas."*
>
> –**Cynthia Clark**, PhD, RN, ANEF, professor of nursing, Boise State University, Idaho, USA, and colleagues

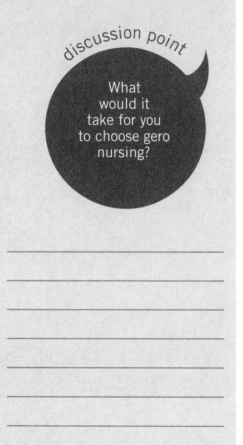

discussion point

What would it take for you to choose gero nursing?

Wanted: Generalist Geriatric-Competent Nurses and Scholars Invested in Teaching Them

by Sarah H. Kagan

Care for aging societies—in our own nation as well as other countries—and support for our aging profession require two fundamental changes in nursing. First, we must constitute a single voice recognizing that baccalaureate-prepared nurses are the single greatest force in improving care of older people. Second, we must transform a mid-20th century curriculum into a national mandate that meets demographic and epidemiologic imperatives.

A singular voice expressing the power of the nurse at the bedside, in the exam room, and at the home allows us to bring that power to the surface in social discourse. While many people recognize the value of nursing, too few understand its necessity or have endured poor care and believe that ours is not a power for good. Our profession commonly distracts discourse with emphasis on advancing education and specialized roles. We imply that generalist nurses are useful but not fundamentally valuable.

However, our projected population and disease demographics suggest precisely the opposite (Institute of Medicine, 2008, 2011). To provide adequate care for older people, the nursing profession must embrace the critical role of the generalist nurse. Nothing replaces the direct care provided by generalist nurses that is essential to the care of older adults. We cannot diminish our capacity to educate generalist nurses in favor of advanced education and specialized training, lest we risk our ability to meet the needs of aging populations.

Undergraduate nursing curricula echo mid-20th century demography when our population was young. To this day, many curricula reinforce antiquated notions of medical-surgical nursing, acute care lacking in transitions, and required pediatric and obstetrical competence. Perhaps no more than 40% of curricula—an optimistic view, based on older data—require geriatric content (Berman et al., 2005), yet all mandate clinical pediatric and obstetrical content. We must reverse this mismatched requirement. Nurses must be competent to care for older adults of varied backgrounds with diverse health needs across all settings of care.

Ensuring that care for older people is a rewarding, exciting option requires that, in finding our singular voice and in reframing curricula, we achieve a celebration of it while recruiting faculty dedicated to teaching the generalist geriatric-competent nurse. Passionate teachers beget excited, interested students and discard ideas of institutional drudgery for intellectual and practical engagement in changing the lives of older adults and their families. Care for older people requires exchanging stereotypical ideas of being old for reinvigorated attention to evidence, action, and outcomes. Our chance to sustain the life cycle of our societies and of nursing is to

What do you think?

_____

_____

_____

_____

_____

_____

_____

_____

_____

It's your turn ... start the discussion!

_____

_____

_____

_____

_____

_____

_____

_____

_____

_____

teach current and future health imperatives and to reward nurses invested in generalist practice and those scholars who invest in teaching our future generalists.

—**Sarah H. Kagan,** *PhD, RN, is the Lucy Walker Honorary Term Professor of Gerontological Nursing and a clinical nurse specialist at the University of Pennsylvania's Abramson Cancer Center.*

References

Berman, A., Mezey, M., Kobayashi, M., Fulmer, T., Stanley, J., Thornlow, D., & Rosenfeld, P. (2005). Gerontological nursing content in baccalaureate nursing programs: Comparison of findings from 1997 and 2003. *Journal of Professional Nursing, 21*(5), 268-275.

Institute of Medicine. (2008). *Retooling for an aging America: Building the health care workforce.* Washington, DC: The National Academies Press.

Institute of Medicine. (2011). *The future of nursing: Leading change, advancing health.* Washington, DC: The National Academies Press.

U.S. Department of Health and Human Services (USDHHS). (2010). *The registered nurse population: Findings from the 2008 National Sample Survey of Registered Nurses.* Retrieved from http://www.thefutureofnursing.org/sites/default/files/RN%20Nurse%20Population.pdf

Question #10:

How Do We Make the Profession as Diverse as the Population for Which It Cares?

Did you know …

"The racial and ethnic profile of the RN population is substantially different from that of the U.S. population," according to the 2008 National Sample Survey of Registered Nurses (HRSA, 2010, p. 7).

We're willing to wager that each and every nurse thinks of something different when he or she thinks of "diversity": race, age, sex, cultural, sexual preference, clinical, educational—the list goes on and on. We're also willing to bet that while many nurses acknowledge the importance of diversity, they don't think there's much they can do to change it.

Nursing needs to make a change if it wants to provide patients of all colors, ethnicities, and religions with quality health care. This change is incumbent on all nurses at all levels, from staff nurse to CNO. To embrace the entire population, nursing must be open and aware. Refusing to recognize cultural differences or being unwilling to change behaviors to embrace nurses of different ages and generations is not an option. Supporting diversity is a professional responsibility.

Some organizations say it would be "good to do," but the smart ones recognize that you *must* do it. It's a leadership issue, a workforce issue, and—most importantly—a patient care issue. Nurses have to look past their own personal preferences and prejudices and do what they need to do to eliminate bias and encourage diversity in every aspect of their practices. Does this sound difficult? Unrealistic? That's why it's time to start the conversation.

Improving Health Care for Hispanics

by Nilda Peragallo

Historically, the United States has taken pride in being considered a "melting pot" of people from many nations and cultures. Unfortunately, this trend of ethnic diversity is not reflected in Hispanic health care professionals in the United States. The U.S. population, fed largely by immigration, will grow to 420 million by the year 2050, according to the U.S. Census. The Hispanic population should be more than 100 million, which is understandable since more than 57% of all immigrants come from Mexico.

Hispanics comprise 13% of the nation's population, and the U.S. Census Bureau projects that this figure will climb to 17% by the year 2020. This expansion, combined with the increasing heterogeneity of the nationalities composing the Hispanic population, underlines the need for accurate information on Hispanics that takes into account their growing diversity.

More than 1.4 million Hispanics are enrolled in post-secondary education, comprising 9.3% of all college students in the U.S. By comparison, 78.3% of students are White and 14.1% are Black (U.S. Census Bureau). The Robert Wood Johnson Foundation (RWJF) has documented how the health care needs of a minority population are uniquely addressed by nurses from the same minority

discussion point

"The U.S. Census Bureau predicts that by 2050, the majority of Americans will be black, Asian, Native American, or Hispanic. In some cities and states, they already represent a majority of the population" (Andrulis, Siddiqui, Purtle, & Duchon, 2010).

By 2050, will the nursing profession still be primarily Caucasian? Why or why not?

Did you know ...

"The workforce is generally not as diverse as it needs to be—with respect to race and ethnicity (just 16.8% of the workforce is non-white), gender (approximately 7% of employed nurses are male), or age (the median age of nurses is 46, compared to 38 in 1988)—to provide culturally relevant care to all populations" (HRSA, 2010, p. 25).

group. However, many Hispanic students cite inadequate secondary education, inability to pay tuition, feelings of isolation, and perceived discrimination.

The RWJF is calling for "greater ethnic diversity" as a catalyst to improve health care for Hispanics. Nearly one fourth of all Hispanics in the United States live at or below the poverty rate and can't afford medical insurance; 32% of Latinos reported their accent led to poor treatment and communication with health care professionals. Hispanics have a higher risk of obesity, alcoholism, smoking-related diseases, sexually transmitted diseases, and a high prevalence of type 2 diabetes mellitus, which is a risk factor for the development of chronic kidney disease (Lopes et al., 2003).

Increasing the diversity of the Hispanic health care workforce will play a critical role in identifying potential health concerns and addressing racial and ethnic health care disparities. Patients feel more comfortable if they can talk to someone who understands their language, beliefs, and values of their culture. Knowing your patients and understanding where they are coming from are both critical in determining a proper course of treatment and outstanding patient care.

—**Nilda Peragallo**, *DrPH, RN, FAAN, is dean and professor at the University of Miami School of Nursing in Florida.*

No Easy Answers to Questions About Increasing Diversity in Nursing

by Maria Elena Ruiz

Many years ago, as a young and idealistic nursing student, I read that Hispanic nurses accounted for approximately 5% of the RNs in this country. Upon graduating from a nursing program in Los Angeles, I remember how proud I felt displaying my nursing diploma. I felt empowered and believed that I, and others in my nursing cohort, would contribute to the rising number of Hispanic/Latino nurses working in diverse communities.

We believed the number of culturally and linguistically diverse RNs would continue to grow. Unfortunately, as shown in both the 2004 Sullivan Commission's report, *Missing Persons: Minorities in the Health Professions*, and the National Sample Survey of Registered Nurses report (HRSA, 2010), this has not been the case. Instead, while this country continues to become increasingly diverse, the health care provider and nursing workforce has been unable to keep pace. Today, 65% of the U.S. population is of white European background. A look at the racial/ethnic breakdown of all RNs shows that the overwhelming number of nurses are white (83%), 5.8% are classified as Asian/Pacific Islander, 5.4% are Black/African American, 3.6% are Hispanic/Latino, and less than 1% are of American Indian/Alaskan Native ancestry. And although the number of men in nursing has slightly

Top 10 challenges

"[To be successful, we must embrace] gender issues in the nursing profession."

—**Erlinda Caster-Palaganas,** PhD, RN, director of the Institute of Management, University of the Philippines Baguio, Baguio City, Philippines

Did you know …

Workforce diversity is up: In 2008, 16.8% of nurses were Asian, Black/African-American, American Indian/Alaska Native, and/or Hispanic—an increase from 12.2% in 2004 (HRSA, 2010).

Recently graduated RNs are substantially more ethnically and racially diverse. Additionally, there are now more male graduates than there were prior to 2001 (HRSA, 2010).

improved, men still only comprise approximately 8% to 9% of the nursing workforce.

The representation of faculty of color in health professional schools was also found lacking by the Sullivan Commission and the American Association of Colleges of Nursing report (AACN, 2004). Less than 10% of faculty in baccalaureate and graduate nursing programs are members of underrepresented minority (URM) groups. In colleges and universities, URM nursing faculty includes 5.6% African American, 1.5% Hispanic, and 1.9% Asian faculty members.

Looking at the types of RN education preparation, we see that RNs from racial/ethnic minority backgrounds are more likely to enter nursing with a bachelor's degree, although they are less likely to pursue graduate and advanced practice degrees. Overall, while slightly more than 83% of all advanced practice registered nurses are White, 6.3% are Black/African American, 4.2% are Asian, and 3.5% are of Hispanic/Latino ancestry.

Drawing from various articles by experienced nursing leaders, as well as from "kitchen talks" in various communities, I have found there are no easy answers to this question. Perhaps more laudable short-term goals are to increase the number of future nursing students, to recruit and retain them, and to graduate nurses who are not only well prepared, but also happy with their nursing experiences. Here are ways we can start:

- Increase the number of faculty of color in academia; they are invaluable mentors and resources not only for students of color, but for all with whom they come in contact.

- Provide opportunities for advancement for faculty and staff of color, including administrative positions.

- Strive for a respectful and culturally empathetic, holistic nursing school environment.

- Develop and support linguistic and culturally diverse curriculums where cross-cultural experiences and service learning in diverse communities are the norm, not an elective.

- Provide enrichment and support for all students, not only for students of color.

- Expand the admissions criteria, whereby life experiences and community service are given equal value to grade point averages and test scores.

What do you think?

_____

_____

_____

_____

_____

_____

_____

_____

_____

Did you know ...

According to the 2008 National Sample Survey of Registered Nurses (HRSA, 2010), RNs from minority backgrounds are more likely than their white counterparts to pursue baccalaureate and higher degrees in nursing. Data show that while 48.4% of white nurses complete nursing degrees beyond the associate degree level, the number is significantly higher or equivalent for minority nurses, including African American (52.5%), Hispanic (51.5%), and Asian (75.6%) nurses. RNs from minority backgrounds clearly recognize the need to pursue higher levels of nursing education beyond the entry level.

- Be open to students and faculty of color; embrace and value them as part of the team.

- Enlist support from various organizations that represent racial/ethnic minority nurses and collaborate with them (i.e., National Association of Hispanic Nurses, Black Nurses Association, etc.), and network with their members. They are already out in diverse communities; learn to partner with them.

–**Maria Elena Ruiz,** *PhD, RN, FNP-BC, is assistant adjunct professor at the University of California-Los Angeles School of Nursing, and is associate director for the Chicano Studies Research Center.*

Top 10 challenges

"[It is essential that we] cultivate a culture of health and healing."

–**Michelle R. Troseth,** MSN, RN, DPNAP, executive vice president and chief professional practice officer, Elsevier

Increasing Diversity to Decrease Health Disparities

by Antonia M. Villarruel

In the last 30 years, there has been a concerted effort and commitment by national and state governments, professional associations, educational associations, private foundations, and others to diversify the health care workforce. Progress has been made toward building infrastructures for diversity efforts that include the implementation of policies to support and sustain such endeavors. As a result, the proportion of racially and ethnically diverse nurse graduates has increased from 12.3% in 1988 to 22.5% in 2008 (HRSA, 2010).

While some might consider a 10% increase in the racial/ethnic composition of the workforce as progress, it has taken 20 years to achieve this gain. Despite these major, multilevel policy and programmatic efforts, the collective impact on diversifying the nursing workforce has been minimal. Closer examination of the proportion of racial/ethnic minorities in roles that require advanced nursing education, which include advanced practice registered nursing and nursing education, are abysmal. For example, among advanced practice registered nurses (APRNs), only 3.5% are Latino and 6.3% are African American (HRSA, 2010).

Increasing diversity in the health professions addresses a social justice and equity issue that helps ensure that all people have an opportunity to enter and advance in

> ## Top 10 challenges
>
> *"[Nurses from other cultures will continue to flock here as] international nurse migration and the subsequent brain drain [continues] in developing countries that can least afford to lose their scarce nursing resources."*
>
> **–Carol L. Huston**, DPA, MSN, MPA, FAAN, director, School of Nursing, California State University, Chico, California, USA

discussion point

Think you can't make a difference? Name three things that you—in your current nursing position—can do today to immediately affect diversity in your practice.

these fields. In addition, the diversification of the health care workforce represents a way in which to decrease the health disparities experienced by both racial and ethnic minorities and socially and economically disadvantaged populations.

So what can we do? There are many strategies that we can adopt: supporting quality public education for our youth, ensuring that children grow up happy and healthy with an opportunity to complete high school, and working within communities to increase awareness and promote careers in nursing are just a few ideas.

As a profession, we have the resources needed to diversify the workforce. Specific areas in which to concentrate efforts include the call for increased accountability and evaluation of programmatic outcomes for those receiving public and private funds to increase diversity; an examination of institutional policies that systematically block racial and ethnic minorities from entering in, progressing in, and graduating from our own schools of nursing; and implementing best practices that facilitate entry and progression.

Two more areas to focus on involve the development of strategic partnerships with minority communities to facilitate interest in nursing and also to work with all nurses to address community health needs. To this end, we must identify best practices in articulation programs between AD and BSN programs, and we must work to disseminate and scale up efforts in schools and communities. We should also pursue similar approaches to increase the mobility of AD graduates to BSN and beyond.

Finally, we ought to engage minority nurse leaders in meaningful ways and support the realization of their full potential to lead in addressing diversity efforts.

There is a long list of what we *need* to do and, importantly, much that we *can* do. The time for action is past: We must act now.

–Antonia M. Villarruel, *PhD, FAAN, is associate dean for research and global affairs, professor, and Nola J. Pender Collegiate Chair at the University of Michigan School of Nursing.*

**It's your turn …
start the discussion!**

_____

_____

_____

_____

_____

_____

_____

_____

_____

_____

_____

References

American Association of Colleges of Nursing. (2004). 2003-2004 salaries of instructional and administrative nursing faculty in baccalaureate and graduate programs in nursing. Washington, DC: Author.

Andrulis, D.P., Siddiqui, N.J., Purtle, J.P., & Duchon, L. (2010). *Patient Protection and Affordable Care Act of 2010: Advancing health equity for racially and ethnically diverse populations.* Joint Center for Political and Economic Studies. Retrieved from http://www.jointcenter.org/hpi/sites/all/files/PatientProtection_PREP_0.pdf

Health Resources and Service Administration. (2010). *The registered nurse population: Findings from the 2008 National Sample Survey of Registered Nurses.* Rockville, MD: HRSA. Retrieved from http://bhpr.hrsa.gov/healthworkforce/rnsurveys/rnsurveyfinal.pdf

Lopes, A.A., Bragg-Gresham, J.L., Satayathum, S., McCullough, K., Pifer, T., Goodkin, D.A., et al. (2003). Health-related quality of life and associated outcomes among hemodialysis patients of different ethnicities in the United States: The Dialysis Outcomes and Practice Patterns Study (DOPPS). *American Journal of Kidney Disease, 41,* 605-615.

Sullivan, L. (2004). Missing persons: Minorities in the health professions. A report of the Sullivan Commission on Diversity in the Healthcare Workforce. Retrieved from http://bhpr.hrsa.gov/healthworkforce/rnsurvey/2008/nssrn2008.pdf

Index

A

Affordable Care Act. *See* Patient
  Protection and Affordable Care Act
aging population, 106107
  generalist nurse, 108110
  geriatrics in curricula, 109
aging workforce, 102103
American Recovery and Reinvestment
  Act, 2425

D

disruptive innovation, 6061

E

ethics, 6676
  end-of-life care, 6667, 7375
  financial parity and, 75
  moral distress, 6976
evidence-based practice
  barriers, 8

benefits, 5
creativity and, 2, 7
definition, 2, 7
facilitators, 8
future of, 58
leadership, 4

N

National Health Care Workforce
  Commission, 3536
National Sample Survey of Registered
  Nurses, 102, 112, 115, 118
Nightingale, Florence, 2, 9, 95, 97
nurse practitioners (NPs), 50, 6061
nursing culture
  bullying, 80
  diversity, 8384, 112121
    ethnic, 83, 115120
    faculty, 116
    gender, 83
    generational, 8589
    Hispanics, 113114

education *vs.* practice, 8182
  working together to improve, 83
nursing education
  associate's degree, 32, 34, 3739
  bachelor's degree as minimum entry,
    30, 3239
  DNP (Doctor of Nursing Practice)
    programs, 42, 44, 48
    standardization for APN, 4850
    vs. PhD, 42
  doctoral graduates, increasing, 4345
  *Essentials of Doctoral Education for
    Advanced Nursing Practice*, 5152
  vs. other health care occupations, 3031
nursing leaders
  developing, 9394
  improving practice environment, 9798
  sharing wisdom, 93
  strengthening profession, 9597

P

Patient Protection and Affordable Care
  Act, 35, 46, 58, 95, 106

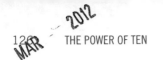
Contributors